Elizabeth Wilde McCor[mick]
approach to recovery from
ing hospital procedure, me
practical advice for the rea
habits, alcohol, smoking, r

She also provides advice,
to come to terms with the emotional consequences of a
heart attack, from the initial feelings of shock, helplessness
and fear to longterm anxieties about the future.

Any breakdown in health is a warning not to continue with
the kind of stressful life which led up to it, often exposing
problems which we have buried beneath habit and routine.
The time following a heart attack can provide an opportunity to reassess our values, relationships and needs.

After a career in journalism and commercial writing,
Elizabeth Wilde McCormick trained as a counsellor, and
took a master's degree in humanistic psychology. Her
special interests lie in the area of stress-related illnesses. She
now practises as a counsellor and therapist in London,
where she lives with her husband and children.

THE
HEART ATTACK
RECOVERY BOOK

A look at the emotional and practical problems
encountered during rehabilitation,
for patients and their families

ELIZABETH WILDE McCORMICK

UNWIN PAPERBACKS
London   Sydney

This revised edition first published by Unwin® Paperbacks, an imprint of
Unwin Hyman Limited, in 1987

First published in Great Britain by Coventure Limited 1984

UNWIN HYMAN LIMITED
Denmark House, 37–39 Queen Elizabeth Street,
London SE1 2QB
and
40 Museum Street, London WC1A 1LU

Allen & Unwin Australia Pty Ltd
8 Napier Street, North Sydney, NSW 2060, Australia

Unwin Paperbacks with the Port Nicholson Press, 60 Cambridge Terrace,
Wellington, New Zealand

British Library Cataloguing in Publication Data

McCormick, Elizabeth Wilde
The heart attack recovery book: a look
at the emotional and practical problems
encountered during rehabilitation, for
patients and their families.
1. Coronary heart disease—Popular works
I. Title
616.1'23   RC685.C6
ISBN 0-04-440061-6

Printed in Great Britain by
Guernsey Press Co. Ltd., Guernsey, Channel Islands

For John

Acknowledgements
to the First Edition

The British Heart Foundation, Action on Smoking and Health, the Office of Population Censuses and Surveys and the International Society for Humanism in Cardiology for their information and co-operation.

The Middlesex Hospital for their co-operation in my visiting and talking to heart patients.

Thanks to all the men, women and families who have talked to me of their experience of heart attack, and who gave their time and their stories while I was involved in research.

A special thank-you to Dr. Peter Nixon for all his support and encouragement in the writing of this book and for his excellent Foreword.

Thanks to Lynn Douet who typed the manuscript and to Ian Fenton who felt inspired to publish it.

A personal thank-you to the friends and colleagues who have offered feedback and support – Anabel Farnel Watson, Ean Begg, Sara Brain, Joyce Varney, Ian Gordon Brown, Penny Butterfield, Renate Fasold and John Andrew Miller.

A very special thank-you to Irene Oxenham, whose friendship, love and tolerance has been behind me for the last thirteen years, and to Barbara Somers, whose wisdom, generosity and example have sustained me at all times.

Preface
to the Second Edition

The Heart Attack Recovery Book was first published in June 1984 with a second printing in January 1985. This 1987 edition contains new sections on high blood pressure; angina; coronary artery bypass graft; exhaustion and fatigue; breathing techniques; and new chapters on counselling heart attack patients and on families and couples involved in a heart crisis.

My original interest in writing this book stemmed from my husband's heart attack in August 1977 and a lot of the book was written from personal experience. To this I have now added a more professional dimension, having consolidated my work as a counsellor and therapist over the last ten years. This time has been marked by the increasing number of people suffering from the effects of prolonged fatigue, exhaustion, depression, and whose coping skills for dealing with stress are sorely stretched. At the same time, people are asking many more questions about how to care for their own health, wanting an holistic approach to health care which embraces body, mind, emotions and spirit, and which also takes in environmental and social factors. Britain still has the second highest number of deaths from heart attack and the British Heart Foundation project a figure of approximately 111,000 myocardial infarctions each year between ages 35 and 69. Many people are looking at their own lives and asking, "Am I living appropriately?" I find it encouraging that people are coming to talk to me, not only because they have had a heart attack and are looking at their process of recovery, but because they feel they may be at risk from heart strain and they want to lessen the risk. The fact that people are recognising the role of personality, behaviour, attitude and psychological make-up in the process of clogging up arteries and pushing up blood pressure, seems to be a breakthrough in general attitude, and a movement away from the literalisation and mechanisation which still dominates much of medicine.

I am deeply indebted to Dr. Peter Nixon and his team at Charing Cross Hospital who invited me to come to their ward rounds and to

PREFACE TO SECOND EDITION

work as a counsellor with their patients. I have been able to absorb their
attitudes towards exhaustion in coronary heart disease, the principles of
anticipation and prevention, surgical treatment and rehabilitation. The
Research Fellows, Miss Jenny King and Dr. Leisa Freeman, have
generously disclosed to me all of their research methodology and results
before publishing the data themselves. I should like to thank Dr. Hywel
Williams, Dr. Sara Pugh and Ashley Conway for their kindness and
encouragement, and Mrs Pam Edwards for her practical help, care and
attention. And I'd like to thank all the occupational therapists and nurses
whose patience, tolerance and expertise makes all the difference in the
world to patients and their families.

Alongside working at Charing Cross Hospital I have been developing
my own counselling and therapeutic work and interest in different
approaches to life management, and in the way illness weaves its way in
and out of our lives and what this means. The meaning of illness, in
particular of heart illness, is a theme that interests me, and I have written
about this and run workshops on this theme. My husband, whose heart
attack inspired this book, remains fit and well, having had a successful
coronary artery bypass graft operation just nine years after his heart
attack in 1977.

I would also like to thank all the men and women who have talked to
me, sharing their stories over this last ten years, and allowed me to
consolidate my knowledge of the work of the heart, both symbolic and
real. I feel privileged to have been able to share these times of crisis and
change, and joyful when a creative movement forward can be found, out
of the chaos, confusion, pain, and fear for the future.

Liz Wilde McCormick
May, 1987

Contents

Foreword

It is almost as if something inside the patient refused to get well until the doctor had really listened to what was wrong and taught the patient to outwit its influence. – Georg Groddeck

PEOPLE ARE NOT naturally equipped to deal with heart attacks. They waste time and lose their way as they muddle through phases of denial, rage, bargaining and depression before getting to grips with one of life's most important problems. Left to their instincts they settle for inefficient ways of coping with the crisis. Some adopt a passive rôle of saintly resignation and others are overwhelmed by despair: each of these courses stifles the urge to set up a happier and less exhausting way of living amongst hard circumstances and difficult people. Many deny the existence of the problem and lose the chance to make the best of themselves.

A large number are driven by panic and rage to struggle mindlessly against the heart's limitations and warnings: wanting to escape they fly like Icarus in uncalculated bursts of excessive effort and then crash, wings burned, forever pushing themselves through vicious cycles of exhaustion and defeat which inevitably worsen the condition of the overtaxed heart.

One of the reasons for these incompetent responses is the fact that the heart attack usually makes its appearance when the individual is drained of strength and resilience by effort which has carried him beyond the limits of his endurance for a year or more. The exhaustion of the body and mind makes it well-nigh impossible to manage the crisis in a calm and sensible way. Blind instinct and primitive responses get the upper hand. The body and mind are not fit, able and ready for the heart's attack. The exhaustion and sense of defeat cry pitifully for withdrawal from the struggle of life for a period of repair and reorganisation, and the conservation of energy, and yet many patients are treated without ever being slept and rested well enough to remove the exhaustion. Nor are they trained to recover fitness, ability and readiness for challenges. Not enabled to recover healthy function they remain ill and become dependent upon pharmacological or surgical palliation of the symptoms of their illness. No one tells them that the heart has an extraordinary capacity for repairing itself and recovering from a heart attack when it is provided with the conditions it needs.

In my opinion, the heart attack rarely comes as a surprise except to those who cannot tell the difference between the first straws and the last straws on the camel's back: not a surprise or an accident but a foreseeable collapse (in mathematical terms, a catastrophe). Not the attack of an enemy from outside but a miscalculation!

It is useful to think of the heart attack as a breakdown of health which has a message: "So far, and no further. Do no go on living as you intend". (Groddeck). Georg Groddeck studied the meaning of illness and his words might have been lines for the heart's addressing the mind. "I gave you far-reaching freedom; since you want to abuse it in internecine quarrels I shall restrict it, and if that does not stop you I shall take it away."

The difficulty of coping with the heart attack in an exhausted condition is compounded by man's inherent inability to withdraw from effort when he has unfinished business on hand, and by the social instincts which make it unthinkable for him to withdraw and conserve his energy while the people who depend upon him continue to need his services.

The ancients had ways for dealing with these impediments to recovery. According to verbal tradition, Athenians who were broken down in health by mathematics or politics went to the Island of Cos to recover. Hippocrates organised the sleep and rest they required and provided them with a relaxing holiday. At the right moment he took them to the gymnasium to be

FOREWORD

made physically tough and highly skilled in assertion. He sent them back when they were well trained and felt like winners!

This Hippocratic prescription of sleeping, resting and re-training was still conventional treatment in Victorian times and the first three decades of this century, and it can still be obtained in Continental Europe. The great English cardiologists, James Mackenzie and Thomas Lewis, certainly put the prescription to good use when they were re-fitting ill and exhausted soldiers for the 1914–18 War, and I sometimes think it was this close understanding of the basic principles of healing which enabled them both to lead vigorous and productive lives for twenty years after the onset of their own angina pectoris.

The 1939–45 War brought in a fruitful and accelerating development of technology but medicine became unbalanced, and heart attacks were treated as if drugs and operations were adequate SUBSTITUTES for the natural cycle of sleeping and resting, enjoying convalescence, and retraining, instead of being ADDITIVES for elegant and precise prescription at exactly the right moment.

The major preoccupations of cardiology just now are to decide how and why the heart attack occurs and how it can best be prevented. From the clinical point of view we probably have enough facts for sensible decisions but research is piled upon research at an astronomical cost to bolster up the causes of the various factions. In ethology this is known as the Concord principle, the name honouring the aircraft upon which we spent millions to justify the magnitude of the previous investments!

The heart attack is far from being the simple result of atheromatous narrowing of the coronary arteries. The arteries may even be normal. In cases where they are narrowed, the narrowings are not detectably different from those of contemporaries who are enjoying good health and continue to do so for years or decades on end. Between the two Great Wars there appeared to be a six or seven-fold increase in heart attacks in one sector of London while the incidence of atheromatous narrowings actually fell. In the nineteen-sixties and seventies it was thought that the major "risk" factors of smoking, raised blood pressure and dietary cholesterol "caused" heart attacks and

xiii

millions of dollars were spent on research programmes which hoped to prove that the "plague of hearts" might be removed by giving up smoking, changing the diet and taking a daily pill to control the blood pressure. Alas, the programmes succeeded in reducing the "risk" factors but their impact on the death and sickness rate from heart attacks was disappointingly small. The reason seems to be that the risk factors are not causal. Furthermore they have a low predictive value: "if we take 100 men with the three major risk markers (smoking, hypertension and raised serum cholesterol) only 8 develop clinical manifestations of coronary heart disease over the next ten years while 92 do not. Conversely, most previously fit patients who developed coronary heart disease while under the Seattle Heartwatch programme had no conventional risk factors on entry". (Editorial, British Medical Journal, 1977, I, 1302.)

Even if they were causal, they could not account for more than 25–30% of heart attacks. The majority of heart attacks have a cause or causes not yet the subject of agreement. It is my belief that the important element is profound and prolonged exhaustion associated with high levels of arousal (rage and despair) which come from the strain of struggling against hard circumstances and difficult people. In exhaustion, the body's self-regulating mechanisms (the homeostasis) become incompetent, and unable to keep the internal milieu in a healthy and stable state: the catecholamine effects of anger and the pituitary-adrenocortical consequences of defeat and despair predispose to arterial damage, atheroma, thrombosis, high blood pressure, and increased blood levels of cholesterol, sugar and uric acid. These catabolic disorders prepare the way for the heart attack which is a sudden collapse of the defences against thrombosis, arterial and arteriolar spasm, shock, and serious disorders of the heart beat. Some people who are exhausted and trapped in high levels of arousal hyperventilate, and the chemical effects of the hyperventilation can aggravate the disorders or precipitate the collapse.

Inherent in this belief is the feeling that the exhaustion and arousal which can generate the catabolic disorders of blood pressure and blood cholesterol are also capable of causing unhealthy eating, drinking and smoking habits. In other words, the risk factors can be generated by the same forces which cause the illness. Their presence may well aggravate the illness but their removal cannot cure it. Support for this theory comes from the practice of cardiac rehabilitation. Compelling the exhausted and ill to give up smoking, lose weight and reduce alcohol is an enterprise which rarely satisfies the doctor or makes the patient look well and vigorous, but training for fitness and confidence are commonly rewarded by a drastic and salutary change of habits. Sometimes it seems that the patient changes his habits only when he is ready to reward his doctor for care and attention!

It follows from my beliefs that sleeping well, resting adequately, recovering fitness and learning to tackle life's problems in a positive and successful way are still essential ingredients of an adequate prescription for recovery. They are certainly the elements required for the anabolic (healing) processes of the body to work with greatest speed and efficiency.

Heart attacks occurring in the working period of life in our society are strongly associated with childhood poverty; poor education; growing up in hardship; inadequate mothering; being handicapped by lack of fit with the milieu; lack of appreciation, satisfaction and support; loss of control and prediction; overwhelming effort and defeat; and a life which is lonely and uprooted. All of these associations can be seen as predisposing to the exhaustion and high levels of arousal which cause failure of homeostasis and the catabolic disorders. The direct counter-measures are obviously supportive and educational, but patients find them difficult to obtain in an era when diagnostic testing, palliative drug treatment and surgical procedures hold the centre of the cardiological stage. It is certain that if we cardiologists do not provide the services required the newly-wakened patients of the nineteen-eighties will look elsewhere for them. Perhaps it should be emphasised that training each patient to make the best of himself before embarking on the rigours of life-long drug therapy or open-heart surgery is not antipathetic to surgical treatment. If operation is required, the surgeon is glad to find his subject in a good condition and well-prepared to make a long term success of the procedure.

The nineteen-eighties have brought in a great and growing desire for knowledge that will help people to make the best of their natural resources for prevention, healing and recovery, and I have always thought that the professionals should encourage the processes of education. Times have changed since the early days of cardiac rehabilitation when we were condemned for giving heart patients information which "could only make them anxious". The motto of the British Army's Parachute School is "Knowledge Dispels Fear", and this is a very good motto for the man or woman who is thrust suddenly into a career of cardiac disorder. Elizabeth McCormick has produced an excellent book at exactly the right time and the knowledge she provides is invaluable. It will certainly guide a family away from the incompetent responses I mentioned at the beginning of this Foreword.

I hope that the holders of expensive research grants will come up with useful basic information in time for the author's second edition. I should like to see simple and widely-available scientific rules replacing experience, intuition and 'flying by the seat of your pants' for distinguishing between healthy effort and overexertion, for estimating the cardiac reserves, for calculating the effort of life in various circumstances of happiness and unhappiness, for protecting the heart against the effects of exhaustion and defeat, and for enhancing the recuperative qualities of sleep. Some hope!

I should like to end this Foreword by quoting from *The Healing Heart*; Norman Cousins, International Journal of Cardiology, (1983) 3, 57–65: "For many years, deaths from heart attacks have outnumbered fatalities from all other diseases. That number is now on the decline and will, I believe, decline further with the full realisation, not just by the profession but by the general public, that a comprehensive program of treatment involves both the full utilisation of medical science and the full development of the human healing system. The fact that the belief system can be a vital activator of

FOREWORD

the healing system may serve as an open door to an auspicious
future in medical research and practice."

Dr. P.G.F. Nixon FRCP
Consultant Cardiologist,
Charing Cross Hospital, London.
Founder Member of the
International Society for Humanism in Cardiology.

In this morning assembly I wanted to talk about courage. The word comes ultimately from the Latin through Old French and Middle English. It comes from the word for "heart". It was thought that the seat of bravery was in the heart. It was also the seat of love, and that is no accidental conjunction. Because to love is to be brave. It is to be open and defenceless. Christians believe that Christ showed the greatest love possible by accepting his crucifixion as an act of redemption for the sins of the world. The love turned the defeat into a triumph. But those are just words. When we have to do it ourselves, accept, in love, a great blow, it requires the greatest bravery to continue to be open, receptive and not close up. The only way to achieve it is to realise that to close oneself is to complete the aggressive act, to join in an attack on oneself, attempted murder becomes suicide. We must remain open, even to those who would hurt us. That is why it is not strange that the word for bravery comes from the word for heart.

> *Can you hear me at the back?* Act 1, By Brian Clark
> Amber Lane Press (1979)

THE
HEART ATTACK
RECOVERY BOOK

Introduction

You have bought this book for a reason . . . either you have, or someone close to you has suffered a heart attack and you are wondering where to go from here. You are probably feeling rather worried and anxious, bewildered by all the new information and most certainly stunned by what seems like a cruel body blow. This book offers a 'common sense' approach to recovery from heart attack; it explores the practical realities . . . for example, what do doctors mean when they say "now go home and relax, take it easy" . . . and how do you actually do this if it is completely alien to you; and it explores the more meaningful implications of having a heart attack by looking at the 'B movie' currently playing alongside the obvious conscious reality of living. A heart attack means more than a rude assault upon the body, and exploring what this might be is one of the functions of this book.

It is not a medical book but does contain some inevitable medical facts and tries to look clearly at the mass of conflicting theories currently available about why people have heart attacks and what should be done to prevent them.

It is a book born of personal experience; it incorporates research, interview material, and realisations gleaned from my work as a psychological counsellor and therapist. The belief underlying it is that we break down to break through, and to a more meaningful, richer understanding of life. A heart attack can be an opportunity to look toward life rather than death.

My husband suffered a heart attack in August 1977 while we were on holiday. I had been a writer and journalist for several years but was just starting work in the psychological field. I was shocked to find how few resources I had to draw on to help me support him at this time. There were so many questions that remained unanswered . . . how much should he try and do and how soon? There were so many medical opinions, which one should we listen to? He was given leaflets on what not to eat which would conflict with a report we read in the newspapers; one doctor would put him on a drug and another take him off it. The typed list of things not to do, including the cryptic sentence "If you should feel sexually aroused please ring your doctor", which we were given as he left hospital, was perhaps a brave attempt to get some sort of order out of chaos, but bore no relation to the reality of the man who needed a suitable framework in which to begin his convalescence. At no time, even after our return to England, did anyone refer to the mass of emotional feelings he was struggling with inside: the numbness of shock, the fear of suddenly suffering more pain or disability; the loss of identity, the insecurity of the future, the reasons why. No-one spoke of the fear or the nearness of death. And throughout this was the question for me . . . how was I to help and support him in the most loving and constructive way at the same time as dealing with my own fears and anxieties and not passing these on to him? I was lucky enough to be surrounded by thoughtful friends and colleagues experienced in dealing with loss and crisis who gave me a great deal. But in the end I was alone and it was in this loneliness that the seeds for this book were revealed.

There seem to be several distinct phases to the experience of heart attack. The initial feeling is one of shock; shock that on an ordinary day when thoughts and energies are about immediate practical tasks ahead, we are plunged within seconds into the more thought-provoking, fundamental matters of mortality and human frailty.

The second feeling is one of helplessness . . . "How am I going to cope?" The sufferer is tied by his (or her) body to a hospital bed, every basic need being met by others; his (or her) spouse, friend or family may think "how can I keep my job/run the house . . . look after the children, keep friends and relatives informed, make all the decisions that he usually does, understand the car . . . cooker . . . bills . . . office, know what to say to all the others in his life . . . as well as going to see him in hospital or looking after him at home?"

The third feeling is one of anger. "Why me? . . . why does all this have to happen to me, to us . . . just as things seemed to be OK . . . what have I/we done to deserve it all . . . it's not fair . . ." and on top of anger comes the impotent frustration of not being able to do anything about it but go with it. For the person closest to the heart attack sufferer there are often angry feelings covered immediately with guilt and shame for feeling angry when someone else is suffering.

Feelings of shock, helplessness and anger all intermingle with each other from about the third day after a heart attack when the initial profound shocked numbness has begun to wear off. The intensity of them varies from person to person and has a lot to do with the relationships with people and with life at the time. This is a time when, if things had been lurking or brooding under the surface, they present themselves more powerfully. Any relationship difficulties have to be faced, loneliness becomes more acute, dissatisfaction with job, housing or environment seem more acute. When we look more deeply into the personal meaning behind a heart attack we may find that this is what it was all about. It is important that we do not hide or repress the strong feelings at this time but find a way of experiencing and dealing with them, anchoring them so that they may serve a useful purpose. Repressed angry feelings tend to reveal themselves negatively . . . in sullenness perhaps, cynicism, quick cruel remarks or jokes, oblique criticism or in displaced activities such as overeating, overwork, or playing a martyrish rôle.

After these initial reactions there comes a long period of readjustment. Life is not the same again. Something has changed, shifted. If you are in a marriage or relationship there is often a reversal of rôles for a while and an opportunity to rebalance the working of such a relationship, if this is needed. A heart attack often forces people to express needs which they have never been able to acknowledge to another before. For some men it is the first time they have been able to express their feelings, the first time they have been vulnerable or their wives seen them vulnerable. Often people try and deny having had a heart attack and carry on just as if nothing had happened; partners can collude in this too by hurrying things along in order to "get back to how things were before". This is a natural defence against change, but it is important that the fear of change is looked at . . . what do we really fear might happen to us if we change? What is it we are hanging on to? If you are alone in life with very little that is meaningful around you, the aftermath of a heart attack is a painful time of realisation . . . but it may be the first time you have had to fully acknowledge to yourself your vulnerability and frailty, the fact of your mortality and your need for human contact; your heart attack has made this statement for you to the outside world. It may not be the way you would choose to communicate your needs, but something inside you could not wait for you to speak out and acted for you. The time of rehabilitation can be used to explore some of these issues.

A heart attack loosens the soil in which we have planted ourselves and it throws up both the old weeds and new seeds. Like most other profound human experiences, it is what we make of it, as much or as little as the energy we are prepared to put into it. This book offers some ideas about how to use this time creatively so that your life is more highly valued and lived fully in a new and enlightened way.

Chapter 1

Hospitalisation

a. Shock

So it's a heart attack . . . something that happens to other people, that you hear about from friends or read about happening to people whose names interest the newspapers. This time it is you or someone close to you and you can't believe it. All you know most probably is that you have been plummeted from your ordinary life into a totally new world: that of medical terminology, medical decisions, hospital procedure, a sea of new faces, explanations, words, and indefinable emotions coming unexpectedly in great waves. We all act differently under stress and in emergency but it is amazing the number of people who say "I can't think how I managed, or what kept me going", "something just took over", "I went on automatic".

After a heart attack has been diagnosed and the patient is admitted to hospital the main task is to create a situation in which the suffering body can get on with the job it has to do. The body has amazing natural healing processes which begin to take over from the second that the equilibrium of bodily functioning is disturbed. In childbirth, a woman has to learn to 'dissociate' in order to give all the energy she possibly can to the uterus to complete its work. She does this by concentrating on the other parts of her body, relaxing them consciously at the same time as giving her energies to her uterus. After a heart attack the heart needs energy to sort itself out, sometimes aided by drugs or surgery, but often by itself. Anxiety, fretting, worrying, fighting the process, are all ways in which this energy can be dissipated. The path through the early shock of this experience is to concentrate on the heart sufficiently to aid it rather than act against it.

Here is an exercise which might be offered to someone who has had a heart attack and who is conscious and in pain. As a helper and supporter, you could use all or just parts of the following, as appropriate:

Imagine that you are floating on water or on some soft supportive substance you like. Every little bit of you is being supported from the top of your head to the ends of your toes and fingertips . . . actually picture a soft carpet or cushion, gentle foam or warm water, your favourite colour, and you are totally free to let go, to relax, to be supported completely. Begin with the tips of your toes and go through each part of your body in turn, consciously tightening and then letting it go. Remember the places which usually hold tension . . . the knees, buttocks, neck, jaw and shoulders. When you get to the heart area, imagine that this is the part of you that's just gone in for repair. It's hurt, damaged in some way. It often helps to find an analogy . . . it's like my car engine when the points are clogged up . . . it's like a winged bird, a bruised elbow, whatever your personal imagination brings you. Imagine, then, what this particular symbol most needs to aid its recovery . . . a greater flow of fluid, blood maybe . . . imagine this flowing from your veins and arteries; concentrate on this process so that it seems one in which you are actively involved. Maybe the picture you get is that your heart needs rest and peace. Give this to it from your imagination . . . maybe a summer holiday you've always wanted, a place alone to read or write or plan a garden . . . make a secret place for yourself where you can go and contemplate how you might give some peace to yourself, look upon it as a restorative, nourishing time. Whatever images come up for you, trust them, let your mind take them where they will, and if nothing happens just let your mind wander where it will from its cushion of comfort supporting you underneath. Whilst the medical facilities carry on around you, ministering to your body carefully and efficiently, carry yourself off into a world of the imagination, giving yourself from inside all the rest, nourishment, energy, love, forgotten joys.

The shock of those nearest and dearest to someone having a heart attack is often delayed because of having to be the active ones in coping . . . once again it is amazing how often hidden talents of competence and order come to the forefront in an emergency, and the ability to keep calm . . . often people say . . . "it was a question of act now, keep cool and calm, do what has to be done . . . and feel it all later".

Once you have satisfied yourself that your heart attack patient is in the right place and as comfortable as can be in the situation, it's a good idea to find a place to have a quiet moment to yourself, to evaluate your position . . . you have probably left a house or a job or children in a hurry and these situations will be weighing on your mind. You will wonder who you need to contact and how soon; what to say. You will probably not be able to take in many medical details at first and there is no reason why you should. It is quite enough to tell people that Sue or Alex has had a heart attack and is in hospital or at home. Remember that you are in shock yourself and may easily be thrown off-balance. When people say, as they so often do when they are not directly involved . . . "what treatment is he having . . . what drugs are they giving him?" you need to have planned to say that you will let them know all the details later on and that you are a bit pressed at the moment. Naturally friends and relations are concerned, but they can ring the hospital themselves if they wish. When people are first told of someone's illness on the telephone they often react by wanting to know everything all at once in a rush of worry and concern, trying to get the complete picture so that they can feel in touch, understandably; but it can feel like the Spanish Inquisition. I remember responding with some alarm when one of my husband's relatives asked me if he was on a monitor . . . I didn't know what a monitor was then, and we were on an island where medical facilities were somewhat primitive (only one thermometer to go around fifty people) . . . but it made me anxious and I thought . . . "Oh help, perhaps he should be . . . perhaps I should make a fuss, try and get him one". So you need to limit what you give out at first. Be firm and perhaps ask well-meaning friends and relatives for practical help: perhaps you need help with collecting children, taking the dog out, meals, or looking after other relatives. Letting people help at a time like this is an important part of sharing the load and the more people who feel they are involved, the better.

When you eventually do get home and the house is still and quiet after all the drama, find a comfortable place to sit down. You will probably feel exhausted and upset . . . it is often best at times like this to be wary of the desire to bustle about and be busy so that you don't have to face your thoughts or feelings. Some people say "if I began to think about it, I couldn't bear it" . . . "if I start crying I'd never stop" . . . I believe it to be useful to give vent to one's pent up feelings rather than store them up so that they burst out suddenly and inappropriately. Tears are natural, healthy and useful. Let them fall when they are triggered off by a memory, a phrase, a photograph. This is *your* time, when your cheerfulness, efficiency, stiff upper lip, duty, are not needed. There should be a portion of the day when you have this time for yourself during this crisis, however long it goes on for. This is your let out, your freedom place where you say, shout, rage, write, all the things you have been unable to express during the day. It is amazing how clearing a process this can be and how energising it can be for the next twenty-four hours. Go towards whatever you find soothing . . . something highly personal . . . a pet, a piece of music, a particular friend or relative. I used to return to the house of one of the hospital nurses where I was staying and arrange flowers, and I walked everywhere. These little rituals became very important. Use them for yourself consciously saying "this is one for me".

If the person you are close to is a wife or husband, intimate friend, lover, daughter, son, mother, it's likely that you'll be more worried about them staying alive than anything else. The odds are in their favour that if they have survived a heart attack so far, they will pull through and recover. Keep willing them to pull through this crisis. Have faith that they will. No doubt you will not be able to stop thinking about them, about their health and any events that led up to the heart attack. You will probably go over all kinds of details, eating habits, doing too much, getting into debt, not having a proper holiday, etc. Try not to think "if only . . ." or "I wish we hadn't . . ." or "I wonder if I'd not gone to work" or ". . . gone to work" . . . or "we'd not bought this big house and taken on a large mortgage . . .". Save the working out reasons why it has happened for later on when you are discussing together what things in your lives should be changed, for when you are re-evaluating your position and putting your priorities into some order of merit. It is true that it is comforting to have a reason why or to blame some external factor when things go wrong, but it really does not help at this time. What has happened has happened. You have no choice but to accept it, and to try and do so without the complication of bitterness, rancour or the lip-curling "I told you this would happen if you didn't stop . . .". Although you may not be able to appreciate it at first, you do have in front of you the opportunity to make a better, healthier life. You have the chance to really see what is important, to feel into what is needed now, to answer honestly all the nags that you have kept underground or which have perhaps been rubbing silently away at your happiness. The shock of being near to death may jolt you into a realisation of how precious is what you have between you, and if this has been camouflaged by the weight of years and responsibility, then the present crisis will reveal it.

So, instead of nagging at the reasons why, just at this moment, spend a bit of time thinking about the person you have just left in a hospital bed . . . what are they like . . . what is it like for them to be confined to immobility? Suddenly their world has changed from being active and full to being passive, almost like a baby again . . . being fed and washed, turned over perhaps, every move recorded and analysed by a team of strangers. How will they react do you think? With frustration, tearfulness, withdrawal, overjollification? They most probably will be drugged with tranquillisers such as VALIUM or ATTIVAN, or on painkilling drugs such as PETHIDINE or MORPHINE.

Rest and peacefulness are crucial to the immediate post heart attack period, but inevitably moods and anxieties reach the surface in between sleeping and resting. These can be activated by seeing visitors, receiving letters and cards, telephone calls. If you are close to someone and can protect them from too many visitors, too many calls or letters from wellwishers, too soon, so much the better . . . hopefully for the first week your patient

9

will be so cocooned in the hospital safety that he will not fight to deny the whole thing or to demand that his office or family be summoned to his bedside. Visitors can be very tiring. A heart attack is a highly charged emotional experience and raised pulse rates or blood pressure dangerous. My own husband was denied a television set for his entire stay in hospital for this very fact of over-stimulation. But you, as the closest person, need to take responsibility for checking these things out . . . you know what sort of news or people are likely to trigger off anxiety or fear and you need to be able to take charge. It might be a new experience, and challenging, but a very important part to play, and you can control this stage of recovery, certainly much more than later on.

It is very important that he rests and sleeps as much as possible, and that his mood is kept relaxed and free of strain. The drugs will assist this state, but in between bouts of sleeping and resting he may find that all his thoughts and worries come alive, are stimulated by seeing other people, or receiving messages and flowers, reminding him of a world outside from which he has been forced to withdraw. These times can be very upsetting. Somehow you have to strike a balance between letting him know that his friends and relatives care very much about him and wish him to get better soon, and meeting this knowledge with the understanding of how threatening the outside world can be when you are cut off inside a hospital bed. Even if he is at home you will need to monitor his calls and visitors. In this aspect the buck stops with you. You are the person who knows what news and what person are likely to trigger off the most adverse reaction and it is within your control to handle this situation, remaining friendly and tactful to callers who might disturb the peacefulness. I know of one patient who, on the third day after a severe coronary, received a telephone call from his daughter. She was very upset by his illness and she made no attempt to hide it. The sound of her tears at the other end of the line caused him such agony that his blood pressure shot up twenty points, his chest began heaving up and down with his own sobs and it was some time before he got over it. "Daddy, Daddy, please don't die" the wretched twenty-four year old girl wept over the phone. Unfortunately, not everyone is sensible in these circumstances and you just cannot take chances. A card from the office, however well-worded and concerned, will trigger off anxiety and fear. It could be wiser to leave his cards and well wishes until the third or fourth day after the attack, and certainly to leave most visitors until much later. Ask him who he would like to see. Most probably he will want to see the people who are his real friends, with whom he feels comfortable and can be himself, where he doesn't have to put on an act and perform a part. It is a very revealing time. In some ways it is easier only to allow family to see him at this stage, rather than one person and not another . . . it is amazing how competitive people can be under the disguise of wanting to cheer somebody up and to be the first there.

b.   Cardiac Ward Procedure

It is unlikely that at this stage the coronary patient will be in a position to take in all the details of what is happening to them and their heart. When they are feeling more alert, and this varies a great deal between different people, and feel ready to absorb information, it is extremely important that they do spend some time thinking about what questions to ask. But early on in the illness, family and caring friends can get a strong picture about what has happened and what treatments are taking place.

Once inside a hospital you are on someone else's territory with a given set of rules and hierarchy. It's very important that hospitals are run this way but there's no reason why this kind of 'shutting out' power should intimidate you. You can make a nodding acceptance to the structure of others but not get pulled into it so that you feel depersonalised. Doctors and nurses aren't gods, even if they sometimes behave like them. They do tend to be very busy, especially in places like intensive care units, coronary care units and cardiac wards. It's best to try and choose the appropriate time to ask questions – find out when the best time is and who the right person would be to answer questions. Many hospital personnel who come into contact with patients are not able to answer – technicians, students, cleaners, physiotherapists. They may have their own view and individual scare story or piece of old wives' tale, but this is unhelpful and may even be alarming. So choose your time and be prepared with intelligent questions. Chapter 3 gives some medical information about terms, equipment, physiology, etc. and a suggestion of what might be useful to ask. All you need to know is what you are going to have to carry on at home, what are the likely effects of drugs or treatment, what is the area and extent of damage to the heart.

All hospitals have their own routine and you'll soon get familiar with this. For the patient in intensive care or a coronary care unit, time seems like an endless series of bodily monitoring and whispers. The most, and best, a friend can do is sit by their side and hold hands. They may not seem to notice you but your presence *will* be felt. There is much scientific evidence to show the good effect of human caring on the level of blood pressure arousal in a patient in intensive care!

Most units dealing with cardiac emergency will let one close relative be there and many more doctors and nurses are beginning to recognise the value of a loved one's presence during this crisis stage. There may be a drip feed in the arm giving a transfusion of glucose or saline to feed the body's shock and loss of fluids. Probably electrocardiographic equipment will be strapped to the chest, leading to a monitor which will show the heart beat and pulse rate and which will be watched constantly by a nurse, either in the same room or in another 'monitoring room' where all the monitors of the unit are watched. There may be all kinds of strange looking equipment in the room, which will be bare and sterile and possibly like the space capsules that take people to the moon. There may be a catheter going to the bladder and emptying it of urine into a plastic bag which will hang on the bottom rung of the bed, or an oxygen mask may be used to help breathing. Blood will be taken from the arm to go for laboratory tests. Most likely, injections of pain-killing drugs will have been administered, making the patient rather dopey, sleeping most of the time, maybe muttering a bit. As the relative or friend, just being there is all you can do – reaching out from your own heart as best you can. You might take a book or some handiwork, but sit there as long and as often as you can. I remember reading *The Good Earth* by Pearl Buck as it poured with monsoon-type rain outside and my husband turned all the colours of the rainbow – yellow, white, grey, blue, chalk, and his skin looked alternately parched and loosened. I sometimes look at him now, especially when he's tanned and laughing, and am amazed at the chameleon the body has to be in one lifetime.

Time in intensive care can be two or six days. After this the various equipment contraptions are removed and the bodily functions manage on their own. Most coronary patients do not get out of bed for one week and don't walk more than a few steps for ten days. Then it's a question of pacing. Twenty, thirty, forty steps at a time. It's amazing how tiring even getting out of bed and sitting in a chair has become. But it's a question of slowly, slowly. Things are still at an early stage. It's much more a case of doing, being, than talking, probing or expectations. It is all new ground. Along with it may come difficult, painful realisations and the provoking presence of limitations, but you can only go with what happens – using the material as it is revealed before you. It helps not to have expectations at this stage.

Goals? What happens is that you rejoice at the smallest (but also the greatest) – walking a few steps; walking a few steps without pain; walking to the end of the ward; the end of the corridor; down the passage. Going to the window to breathe the air. Having a bath; going to the lavatory in private; putting on clothes; going in a car; seeing life outside again with the eyes of one who very nearly didn't; seeing home; getting into your own bed; walking around your own garden. Talk about being reborn . . .!

Most coronary patients spend two to three weeks in hospital, but this depends on the individual case and what treatment has been determined. You will be surprised at how much you do take in of medical detail during this time. What in the beginning seems a confused nightmare becomes familiar and able to be understood. As questions arise you need to write them down and have them ready for the appropriate time when you see the doctor or cardiologist who can answer them. How much you want or need to know depends on the kind of person you are. It is not necessary to know complicated medical detail unless you are specifically interested and intend to do a lot of hard reading. Remember that a little specialist knowledge gleaned out of context can be very dangerous. But you do have 'rights' – you have a right to know what people are doing to your own body, and to know what is happening.

c. *"It hasn't happened"*

Sometimes when a really big event occurs in our lives we cannot take it all in. It is too big, too enormous, too frightening to contemplate. We might feel that to take it in would mean to be overpowered by it, weakened in some way, even reduced to nothing. The way in which we defend ourselves from these frightening thoughts is to deny that anything important has occurred, or dismiss it with a "just a little pang in the heart . . . better in a day or two" . . . "it's all that summer pudding I ate". Some people try and rush through "getting over" what has happened to them so that they can "get back to normal". I knew one very successful, ambitious man who found it impossible to relax after his heart attack. He refused sedation, insisted on a telephone in his room so that he could talk daily to his office, kept getting out of bed when he had been advised to lie still and busied himself with note taking, reading, organising all the people around him. He tried to carry on as if nothing had happened. He appeared to recover quite quickly from his first heart attack, priding himself on his fitness and "guts", but succumbed to another, much more serious attack within three months when he was forced, tossing and turning, to contemplate his situation.

Let's ask ourselves . . . how often have I carried on as though nothing had happened even though I felt at death's door . . . how many times have I refused to listen to anyone even though

I knew deep down they made sense . . . how often have I struggled against the feelings or wishes of my body; indeed, how much am I in touch with what my body needs . . . do I try and steamroller over it feeling it to be a nuisance, simply a time-waster? How much of a gap is there between that 'deep down' feeling that 'knows', and the over conscious "I must" . . . "I ought" . . . that drives us on: in psychological terms the gap between the 'self' and the 'ego'. Until we can get some sense of these two aspects of our way of operating as human beings we tend to be at the mercy of ego consciousness, driven on by well learned patterns at the expense of our more subtle inner awareness. It is very hard for our families and close friends to stand by and watch us in our denying carapace whilst our bodies struggle for life. Understand it as they may, they feel helpless and terrified. It is hard, too, to know what help to offer, what support to give. Somehow a way needs to be found to help the unburdening of what it is that gets in the way of accepting that after a heart attack it is the body which has claimed total attention, and that the external world must wait . . . otherwise there will be no body and no external world. Some hospitals have trained cardiac social workers, occupational therapists, nurses and doctors who may offer a bridge into discussion. This is not the time for deep analysis of fundamental behaviour patterns, but the beginning of the possibility of talking about oneself in a new, more personal, way. Contemplation is necessary before any of the benefits of relaxation or meditation are likely to have any effect. There is no point in paying lip service to relaxation classes if we go along with reluctance and half an eye on the clock. Relaxation becomes then just another thing to learn and master and get through and will have no benefit whatsoever. The same goes for meditation techniques or yoga . . . there can be little real help in learning these if the attitude behind it is of just doing it passively as though one were taking a pill and expecting it to work wonders for one. There really needs to be a measure of belief in the experience of letting go sufficiently to go with what happens.

Let's look at what we might be defending. Is it a fear of acknowledging feelings? Do we imagine that if we take a look at the emotional feelings inside us we will be pulled into some kind of boggy ground that will be worse than lying in a hospital bed? Are we afraid it will be like opening Pandora's Box? Do we fear that if we start talking about our feelings it will make us weak? And that if we are weak we will be useless and no one will want to know us? Or that we won't know what to do with such feelings if we do come across them, and this helplessness and confusion will take away our power to live and to make things happen? Also we can be afraid that if we begin to acknowledge feelings we might not like ourselves and what we see. There is the right time and the right place to begin looking at ourselves meaningfully and deeply. No one can force us into 'self-knowledge' and enlightenment cannot be bought or learned from text books. But life does throw up opportunities which we avoid at our peril. I discovered from talking to coronary patients that about 80% had had several accidents during the six months preceeding their incident. My own husband was nearly killed by a helicopter blade in May, dislocated his shoulder while water skiing far out at sea in June and had a heart attack in August. Some would dismiss these events as mere coincidence, but I sense there is more to these things than this; that the force of life itself is offering us a warning, encouraging us to stop and contemplate, giving us an opportunity to look at our lives more fully. Some people do have the Saul on the road to Damascus type of experience which changes their lives, but most of us face more everyday ordinary crises which offer us both danger and opportunity . . . books, films, people, overhearing a conversation, the death of a friend, accidents, illnesses, or even a change in modern dress or music, may sow a seed which takes us on an inward journey.

So what then are our particular worries and idiosyncrasies . . . what do we fear most, what is it that the heart attack has brought to our attention that we can avoid no longer . . . our job: do we like it, is it too big or too small for us . . . is someone standing over us or getting in our way that frustrates or angers us; our relationships: do we have any that are important or do we feel oppressed by them, suffocated, choked . . . are we lonely or unhappy? Do we worry about money, about the future, about growing old, dying? Do we worry because we fear we will never get anywhere in life; is there something that we have been unable to face that our present illness will force out into the open? Is our present illness a kind of 'permission' to speak out about our needs? There may be no immediate solution to our problems but to be able to share them, to unburden oneself of them to someone freely without fear of judgement or criticism is an immense relief. At this stage it is the first step to getting better. Some problems have no solution and it's important to accept this consciously rather than fretting over difficulties carried as a secret burden. Once we face our dilemmas more consciously we also release more energy, all the energy that it took to keep those dilemmas under lock and key, and once this begins to happen we can begin to feel into the wisdom of allowing other parts of ourselves to speak out their needs. If we come up against a really serious problem in our lives that we do not even dare to whisper about just yet, we need to begin to contemplate at this stage and look at it in more detail when we are much stronger, during convalescence. I shall be returning to this subject in Chapter 2 under the heading "*Why, and what does it mean?*".

For now, begin by pondering about these things. One thing is sure, if we can direct all the energy some of us give to our motor cars, ideas, money, jobs, fashion, we have a powerful energy source for recovery and can channel it into our needful spirit and body. Just as negative emotion can produce negative symptoms like depression and feelings of hopelessness so can positive emotion produce positive symptoms*. A person who refuses to acknowledge that their body is just as significant an organ as that which he places highest does as much damage as if he had taken an overdose.

d.   Breathing

Sometimes when we've had a shock or have a period of anxiety,

---

* *Power of Mind* by Adam Smith

it affects the way we breathe. We may 'forget' to breathe or breathe shallowly from our upper chests, taking in great gulps of air to compensate every now and then; sometimes people find that they are concentrating too hard on breathing, forcing breath in as if they weren't getting enough. Breathing disturbances are a sign that we are under stress, and if we notice this in ourselves or in other people, it is wise to do some breathing exercises three times each day until this time has passed.

BREATHING EXERCISES

Sit with your hand over your solar plexus (abdomen) and practise pushing the muscles in and out so that you can feel them working. Sit straight up with shoulders relaxed but your upper body straight. Breathe in allowing your solar plexus to expand, thus allowing air deep into the lungs. Imagine a balloon being blown up as you fill your whole lung cavity with air. When you breathe out, let the air out slowly, pushing every bit out until your balloon image is empty and deflated. Sometimes it helps to make a noise as you do this, a low grunting from the back of your throat ... this can remind you what you are doing, and those familiar with yoga deep breathing exercises, or who have friends trained as singers, will recognise this sound! Concentrating on breathing properly at least three times each day helps to restore a regular pattern of breathing, so that this healthy breathing becomes more automatic; it also helps us to gain a sense of relaxation and peace. Whilst in hospital, there will be many opportunities to practise breathing properly, and this is particularly important after times of exertion, or stressful encounters with doctors, or family visits. Some nurses and occupational therapists are trained to teach abdominal breathing and relaxation techniques and it is worth asking whether any of the staff attached to the hospital you are in can help in this way.

e. *"Where do I put my thoughts?"*

However defended we are, or however much willpower we

have, being very ill makes us feel vulnerable. How frightening it is, when we have got used to being active, fulfilling a rôle, being identified by a job or relationship, or our learned skills, to find that we cannot call upon these to bail us out of a hospital bed. No amount of money in the bank, property, employees, suitors or friends and family can protect us from the kinds of thoughts which float to the surface of consciousness whilst we lie flat on our back. Later our learned skills and acquisitions from life will play a very important part in our recovery.

Sometimes we use our external life to put a stop to irrational thoughts. We plan and plot what we are going to do when we get home, we make promises to ourselves, and this is a great comfort. But in between these links with reality odd thoughts pop up, often in the dream-like state between being awake and asleep and vice versa. It is not uncommon for memories from long ago to be stirred and what appear to be irrelevant connections with the past. Also feelings of childishness and dependency, frustration and fury may be aroused from the fact that we are rather in a babylike position again, tied to a hospital bed and being nursed through all our bodily functions. A man's family may be alarmed to find him sulky and petulant but it is even more alarming for the man himself . . . both to experience these primitive feelings and to be seen to experience them. Not the man a woman thought she married and not the father the children tackled in football.

This regression does not last long unless there are more serious underlying psychological problems. But all the irrational thoughts and feelings of this time are very important, part of the 'B movie' that I mentioned in the introduction.

I know of a man who became very irrational and childlike after his heart attack. He worked as an accountant and was very strict with himself and his family. It was a great shock to see him crying and pouting, banging his fists on the pillows and snarling at his wife when she tried to comfort him. But he had a wise daughter who came and sat with him, knitting, while she told him stories about her day at school and her life in the drama club. He became lulled by the tone of the story telling and fascinated by the colours and weaving of the knitting, the ritual of clicking needles and repeated stitches. One day he idly picked it up whilst he was telling his daughter a story. She left it with him when it was time to go home and he fiddled with it, more interested in the colour and the weave than anything, but enjoying the absorbtion of the repetition of the rows. While he 'played' with the knitting, teaching himself, he thought about his childhood. He remembered his grandmother and her stories, her knitting, sitting by the fire hearing her talking, her laughter, watching the flames dance and listening to the click of the needles and the tick of the old clock. Here he had felt very safe, a feeling of "this is how it ought to be", a promise for the future that had in his life somehow not been realised. He thought about this time a lot, about what his grandmother had given him. He experienced a 'stilling of the mind' which allowed the frustrated feelings he was struggling with to have a shape in which they might be held, so that other realisations might be woken. Later on when he was sorting out his working life he realised how dull and dry it had become and how much he had lost those other qualities and colours that had been stirred up for him at his grandmother's knee. A chance to put money into a bookshop came up and he took it at once, much to the surprise of his family and business associates. He started a club for writers and began writing himself. He says "those memories I had in hospital and the knitting brought back feelings I hadn't had for years. It seems as though part of me was left behind when I went to boarding school and onto the path following a clever, ambitious father, into the family accounting firm. It would never have occurred to me to question it before, but now I feel as though I have claimed something back that was always waiting in the wings". What he experienced in hospital was a form of meditation which brought deeper memories and thoughts to penetrate the surface. When things are knitted together in this way we acquire more understanding of ourselves, a greater sense of wholeness and much more peace.

There are many ways of 'stilling the mind'. At the hospitalisation stage of the post heart attack period simple ritual containments for our more ragged thoughts are the best. Later on we may want to develop this more and will be able to find the facilities to do so . . . painting or sculpture, writing, planting or creating new kinds of games. For the moment, daydreaming is important, focusing on whatever takes your eye . . . the sky, or, if you are lucky enough to be near trees, on the movement of the leaves. Some people like to use their hands, to doodle, draw shapes or pictures, play solitaire, cards, count matchsticks . . . whatever. At this time the ritual act itself is enough to make a shape for the irrational thoughts and feelings that can emerge. It's useful to have a small rough notebook to jot things down as they come, a 'journal' of this time.

You may feel that this is all too introspective, that you have no use for encouraging ragged thoughts to take shape, and want to get on with reading a good paperback, doing the crossword, making lists, getting better as quickly as possible so that you can go home. All well and good, as long as if and when you do feel the surfacing of unusual feelings or thought patterns you honour them rather than push them away. I believe this aspect of serious illness contains the seeds of what the illness is trying to tell us, and that it is creative rather than self-indulgent or harmfully introspective.

Alongside times for reflection are times we want for reading, listening to music if this is possible, talking with friends or other people in the ward or hospital group. This is not the time for self-improvement, competition or trying to exert ourselves in an impressive way, it is a time when we spend most days in pyjamas and dressing gown being called upon by nurses and doctors to take part in all kinds of tests and note taking, especially if we are in a teaching hospital. There is no other time when we will be so close to our personal barometer of who is and which activities are draining and which nourishing, and it is fascinating to discover who and which falls into each category. We can feel immediately by our tension level and the beating of the heart which people tend to take something away from us and which seem to give us strength and it is vital to get used to this being a guideline. We must limit the stressful contacts and encourage the nourishing ones. Books should be readable and comfortable, whatever that means to us; music should feed the soul, friends warm us.

If you have learned a special way to meditate and are practised at it, you will value this entry into your life at this time. It may be that you already have resources for where to put your thoughts, you may be ready and happy to contemplate your life and what has happened and be asking yourself why now? What does it mean? What do I do next? Some of these questions are looked at in the section at the end of this chapter.

The main focus of hospitalisation is getting physically strong enough to return to our individual worlds. The hospital world is very ordered and focused upon physical wellbeing. Occasionally hospitals are equipped with social workers, nurses and doctors trained in counselling skills, and a small, but increasing percentage use yoga and relaxation teachers, masseurs and trained counsellors as part of their cardiac team. If you have no family or close friends with whom you can talk and to whom you can go to share your rehabilitation time it is a good idea to ask for help from the hospital or Social Services. Most hospitals have a volunteers organisation which can offer support, and the amount the services have to offer varies tremendously from one area to another. When I worked as a volunteer in the cardiac department of the Middlesex Hospital in London, people came in offering lifts, clothes, books, visits and follow-up visits to cardiac patients who had no families or whose families were abroad. Naturally as the time draws nearer for you to leave the hospital you may be nervous about how you are going to cope when the structures you have become accustomed to are no longer there. The gap between the limited, focused if sheltered, life of the hospital ward and the life led before the heart attack may loom large and it is easy to panic and to fill this gap with anxiety rather than slowly going forward finding the middle way or compromise in doing things. This time is about 'being' rather than 'doing' and if we have lived our life by 'doing' it's very hard. It sounds easy when people say "just be yourself", "take it easy", "relax", but we may never have learnt how to just 'be'. When we feel ourselves falling into the trap of panic and agitation because we cannot carry on as we did before we became ill it is good to remember the old Zen philosophy of simply doing the next thing that has to be done – putting one foot in front of the other, doing up buttons, combing our hair, stopping to have four breaths before we climb four stairs. Every step must be taken one at a time, picking up the threads of life as you go along, each stage treated as if it were the most precious thing in your life. It actually is, at that moment.

If you are the one waiting at home whilst someone close to you is in hospital your time can easily be eaten up with worry and anxiety unless you find a way to channel this energy into something more useful. When someone is in hospital you have to believe they are in the best place for the moment and believe in their powers of recovery. Having faith in them, praying for them in whatever way you have of praying, lighting a candle each night after you return from visiting, concentrating on the light and imagining it circling around the one you care for as a kind of protection . . . all these are small rituals which I have seen proved to be effective both for the person at home and the one in hospital. One cannot rationalise why this should be but only have reverence for the power of positive energy and the concept that there are healing forces around us.

You can begin to collect information about the type of heart attack suffered and do as much reading as seems appropriate for you. Some people like to learn thoroughly about what has happened and are keen on collecting medical facts; others have more difficulty in doing this. There are many books about heart attacks and many theories about why people have them and what is the best approach to take. At the end of this book is a list of useful, easy to read books containing basic information written by doctors. More useful still is what you glean from the people treating the patient because this is your main reference point for questions and answers. I say more about this in Chapter 3 on digesting medical information. The time when your spouse or friend is away is also a good time for sorting out and doing all the things you've been putting off. You may find that you are more awake, more alert because of what has happened and that your underlying anxiety wakes you early in the mornings. Rather than lying in bed worrying, use the time by getting up and getting on with some of the jobs that have accumulated. Writing letters perhaps, cleaning out cupboards, finishing off carpentry or sewing, gardening, decorating. Practical work is very useful and very effective even if it's hard to get started.

Chapter 2

Rehabilitation

THIS PERIOD of time after hospital is either spent at home, if this is possible, or in a convalescent home, or at some other place that is agreed upon between you and your doctors. Everybody asks "how long?" And every doctor will give a different answer. Some say at least six to eight weeks before a return to part-time work is attempted, some say three months, or even longer. The best thing is to be guided by the person who has looked after you so far, or the one person of the perhaps many people who have been attending you, whom you feel most drawn towards and trust. Like so many things in life it is a question of trust, and of finding one person who 'feels' right and sticking to that one person and the path of his or her judgement.

I have a friend who, expecting her first baby, was told at the eighth month of her pregnancy that she would have to have a caesarean because the baby had not turned round and seemed set in a breech position. She was extremely disappointed, having wanted very much to have her child naturally. She knew that she could have a second opinion, someone who might offer to try and turn her baby round, but after thinking about it carefully, she decided to stick with her doctor's advice. Her baby *was* born by caesarean section and, in fact, the cord was twisted and knotted in several places. If she had been allowed to go into labour, or the baby had been moved, it would have died.

A heart attack is as personal as having a baby. Many of the decisions are emotional ones and it is in the very intimate decisions about your life that you need someone you believe in.

The wonderful lifesaving, but impersonal, advances of technological machinery tend to draw us away from the value of the unique individual contribution. It is a sad fact that many medical practices and hospitals have become rather impersonalised since the innovation of fast-acting drugs and computerised machinery, and many of the healing arts are forgotten. It is these qualities that you are going to need more than ever during the post-hospital days.

So you leave hospital with pills and messages and a list of do's and don'ts, or maybe you leave without any of these things. Some hospitals in this country now organise rehabilitation programmes. Carol Trelawny-Ross, at the Department of Mental Health, University of Bristol, has been researching into different kinds of rehabilitation programmes available for heart attack patients over the last five years, and has visited many of them. She describes the programmes available as three categories: (a) hospital based, pre-discharge schemes; (b) hospital based, pre- and post-discharge schemes; and (c) community based, post-discharge schemes. The programmes varied considerably, ranging from basic information on relaxation and exercise to a comprehensive programme of groups for daily relaxation, exercise and discussion and support, and occupational therapy over a period of eight weeks. In all cases the post discharge phase begins several weeks after discharge. All of Dr. Peter Nixon's patients leave hospital attached to a 'trainer', an occupational therapist with whom the patient keeps in direct contact via the telephone and regular appointments.

Some community based schemes, started by GPs, nurses, physiotherapists or organised by patients themselves as a 'self-help' group, are extremely successful, offering relaxation and gentle exercise training, training in breathing techniques, group discussions for patients and for patients and their partners or family members who are concerned, and a number of visiting specialists to come and talk on various subjects, for example, a sex therapist, dietician, hypnotherapist, physiotherapist and counsellor. Some centres offered leaflets and audio-visual teaching aids as part of their rehabilitation programme for patients and their families.

Carol Trelawny-Ross says

All of those involved in the programes that I investigated were enthusiastic about this aspect of medical care and were unanimous in their appreciation of what was being done for them. All those involved, staff and patients, felt that rehabilitation was an essential part of treatment for coronary patients, not an optional extra.

This chapter looks at some of the main rehabilitation issues in turn. Before we do so, I think it might be a good idea to pause here and have a look at our likes and dislikes, our behaviour patterns and consider what 'type' of person we may be. This will have an important bearing on how we respond to the rehabilitation stage. It could be important, too, for those closest to you to have a look at the personality of the person they are caring for. You probably 'know' only too well but putting a shape to it can often help when things seem to be going not so well. If we can understand why we do certain things or react in a certain way we can be more effective at making changes where these are needed, and it certainly makes us more effective in our communication with others. Looking at what 'type' we are and those types of the people around us also helps us to see how we fit together and where, if any, the sticky areas might be. Jungian psychology outlines four main types, but of course all of us are a mixture of all four, one or maybe two more dominant than the others and one or two a bit lacking. No one can be pigeonholed into one category but it is interesting how often people say "Oh, I'm the emotional type" . . . "he's always thinking it all out" . . . "he's the keep fit fanatic" . . . and so on. Here, then, are the four main 'types':

THE INTUITIVE TYPE

This person is good at 'hunches' and using his 'nose'. Intuition is often deemed a woman's prerogative but many men show their powers of intuition by backing good business deals, knowing which men and women to employ, winning at cards or horse betting, or having a strong sense of purposefulness in their lives that they cannot put into words. Intuiting is often confused with feeling. Feeling sure about something, sensing that something is wrong, are examples of intuiting. Such a person can often be maddening to live with because they cannot really tell you anything. They may say they are going to go out to buy some wood to make cupboards and come back hours later having met someone they knew and bought a motor launch instead. The motor launch will turn out to be the best thing that ever happened. Intuitive types are often good with children, have a vivid imagination, are good at telling stories although they can never tell you where they got them from. However, intuitive people are not always in touch with their bodies. They may try and keep their bodies in control by exercising fanatically, but often this is because they seek a response from the body and are puzzled by its language because it is not one they are most comfortable in.

At the onset of a heart attack, this type of person might say to you "I feel strange . . . I feel that something is going to happen . . ." they may even say, as my husband did "I wonder if I'm having a heart attack" in a puzzled voice before dismissing it thoroughly. They will look puzzled and wonder what strange things their body is going to show them next. Often this kind of person needs someone to help or take over because they will still be puzzling over what is happening when they get to hospital. They may try and ignore their symptoms and get on with something else. They will not be very happy with doctors and medicines and hospital machinery, and will not really want to take an active part in either understanding treatment or taking part in what that treatment is to be. Even when medical terms are explained they tend to forget them and find words of their own. I know one intuitive type of man who, after being told that he had had a myocardial infarction went around telling everyone "I don't know what happened . . . I had some kind of heart fart or something". The intuitive type does, however, have rich resources for developing a creative outlet during recovery. Using those magnificent daydreams and stories they carry around inside themselves they may find ways of expression which astound us: writing, painting, taking up a completely new hobby.

THE FEELING TYPE

This type of person is rather sensitive, although sometimes he may have protected himself with a sharp, brittle surface. He uses his feelings to evaluate the life around him, responds well to other people, has lots of friends, loves to create a loving and happy atmosphere, is good socially and has a lot of strong feelings towards his family. This person is both practical and helpful, takes the initiative when other people need help, leaps in without thinking whenever he recognises something should be done. Feeling types are very good at 'feeling out' other people's situations and understanding them; they are warm people and spread affection and warmth around them. They are not so comfortable, however, with their thoughts. Thinking can often become uncomfortable and stilted, and their attitude can be critical as well as cynical. Because feeling is their main function, they relate everything to their feelings and more often than not do this subjectively. They can be tearful, easily upset and are often unable to communicate what they are feeling. Often feeling types are fairly conventional; they like order and a pattern to things. They can be highly creative on the positive side, and they can be petulant and childish on the negative side.

A feeling type suffering from a heart attack will communicate through his feelings. He will be extremely upset, fearful, anxious and easily overcome with events. Someone in this position might try and deny his feelings in order to be 'big and brave', which is a common occurrence with heart attack victims. A feeling type of man may try and become too much the great thinker in order to remove what he considers a feminine image not suitable for a man. He may try and use the function he is least natural with to try and 'control' the feelings he considers effeminate or too upsetting to his life. He will be the most likely person to deny any idea that he has had a heart attack after the initial fears have worn off. If he has been able to use his capacity for love and feeling in a positive way in his life, he will be able to respond to the caring that comes from his friends and family and to use his crisis positively. Some people of this type will be so much more concerned with the happiness of the people who are looking after them, or for the people on whom they have to depend during illness, that they do not face their own illness without determined help from others. Depression is often something that weaves in and out of the feeling type's life. Once again, their capacity for creativity, for feeling and experiencing beauty and communicating that experience, will be of immense value, as will be their gift of relationship.

THE PHYSICAL OR SENSATION TYPE

This person is in touch with his body, his sensations, his physical needs and abilities. He relates in a concrete and practical way to external objects, he is acutely observant, notices every detail, every texture and substance of outer things. In a room full of people this type of man would be able to tell you how many were there, what they were wearing and possibly how much it had cost. He is uncomfortable with abstract thinking, prefers to stick to the 'facts', and considers matters involving such a thing as intuition a 'mad fantasy'.

Of the four 'types' which I describe in this chapter, the physical type is the least likely to suffer from heart attack because he is used to being in touch with the messages of the body. He is aware of bodily symptoms and deals with them promptly; his reactions are often physical rather than emotional or rational. However, if he is placed in the position of suffering from heart attack, he is likely to tell you what it feels like from a physical point of view. "I'm going to burst" . . . "there is so much tension inside I think a muscle is going to give way/be overstretched" . . . "something's got to give way/be let out/given relief".

This type of person will want to know the facts about what is happening to him and will not rest until he is told. They will be greatly concerned about how long it will take to recover, who will look after their interests while they are away. They will be eager to get well as quickly as possible and will easily see the sense of medication and surgery that will "put things right". They may be difficult to nurse and be impatient with convalescence. If they develop painful symptoms they may be reluctant to discuss them with anyone. They will want to keep them to themselves until they have worked out what they are. They may resent interference in an area where they consider themselves to be superior – after all, who knows that body better than they do? The strong possibility is that they will go and consult their doctor without sharing it. However, after the hospital and during the recovery period this type will have to find a way of relaxing and using this rehabilitation time which will hang heavy for them. Being physically active and 'doing' will not be appropriate at first. Being absorbed in a book, letter-writing, planning a design for the garden, are things they might get on with.

Many physical types have a fine aesthetic sense which can often get buried in busy everyday life. Now is a good time to get in touch with this. Poetry, pencil drawing, just causes, political ideology, are some of the ways of harnessing the aesthetic and the ambitious side of this personality.

THE THINKING TYPE

This person uses his mind to work everything out. When faced with an emotional situation he will gather facts and information about him and think his way through it. Thinking will be his response to most encounters and clarity his objective. He will be a good organiser and effective in government, science, some businesses and in law. Logic is his God. Often such a person is not concerned with subjective issues in life but with the objectivity of the task before him. He is often accused of being cold and over rational, but his acute sense of observation in all matters is only one side to him. When he is ill, one can appeal to his logic, his sense of structure and direction. He is likely to tell you details of the symptoms he has and not the feeling that goes with them. He may concentrate on what he knows of certain symptoms and illnesses or on the ideas he has formulated from this knowledge. He will be the most likely person to respond well to help if it comes in a logical form which he can appreciate.

Where a thinking type may have difficulty is with his

feelings. These may be unaccustomed to being used, as with this kind of person it is the head, or the mind, that rules, and often this kind of ruling does not allow for the expression of feeling. Feeling is nevertheless there, and often piled up and brewing because it is so seldom allowed any expression. Thinking people often surprise us with their passionate declarations. Even though the thinking type will respond well to the reasons for treatment, they may be very uncomfortable with the feelings inside them which are triggered off by the illness. They will not like having the 'props' of their lives removed, the structure threatened. They may try and hide these fears and uncomfortable feelings by having a very sharp tongue and insisting on detailed attention from everyone. At the time of their heart attack, they will be able to be very clear about their symptoms, observant about timing and other details, and they will be able to put all the facts together for their doctor.

The thinking type will probably use their rehabilitation time well, constructively reading and focussing on whatever they decide. They may become moody, depressed because they don't 'think' they are getting on fast enough. Logic appeals to them and if they can see the sense of doing something then they will do it readily. It will be easier for this type to understand exactly what has happened than perhaps some of the underlying reasons. Once they begin to get in touch with these, by getting in touch with their feelings, they will readily understand much more of the meaning of what has happened.

After exploring briefly this typology we might now examine some of the major issues of rehabilitation, placing the person we are or the person whom we know and are helping, into each situation . . . how will I, he or she respond . . . how will I deal with this or like that. Let's bring some of these rather dry and theoretical subjects more alive by placing the person firmly in the middle of them by saying: is this something for me, or him or her?

I debated how much detailed information to go into in subjects like diet and exercise. What I decided to do was give a broad, overall view, outlining some of the more pertinent issues. If any one of these issues appeals to you, and you are wise enough to find out more details – take, for example, food substances containing hidden sodium, not listed as ingredients on the package labels – then I have made a list of books at the end written by experts in their particular fields. Had I attempted to include research details this would have become an unwelcome tome, almost unapproachable. As you read through this chapter, examine how much you are involved in each subject, how important it is to you. Are your habits healthy and creative ones or is it time to think about change? In many of the sections, I talk about establishing 'lifelines' for the future; a set of habits, learnt now in this rehabilitation stage, which create a safety net under you for the coming years; habits which actively work together to give you a happier, healthier life.

a. Exercise

The amount of exercise you can take depends upon the heart rate you are advised not to exceed at this time. None of us know how much exercise we may do and its effects upon our heart until we learn to take our pulse before and after exercise. If you have been advised to keep your heart rate below 110, then you must see how far you can go, or how many stairs you can climb before reaching this rate. Pulse levels do vary from one day to another. You might find that you can walk ten stairs and move your pulse from 80 to 100 on one day, and the next day it might be fifteen stairs or five. Start with your resting pulse and keep a record of this so that you can get some idea of what your normal resting pulse is. In the early days after a heart attack, this will fluctuate a great deal, but when you are home and beginning to get back into an exercise routine, knowing what for you is a starting off pulse is very important. When you have become used to taking exercise you may find that your resting pulse drops, as your heart requires fewer beats to do its work. If you go out for a walk, take your pulse after the first five minutes and see how many points it has risen. If you are getting near to your limit, rest where you are – by sitting down or leaning upon a gate – until your pulse has dropped and you are ready to go on again. This way you can keep up with the body's requirements rather than push your body to fit external goals and targets. Some people find this method of exercise tedious at first, but as you get used to it you will find it rewarding in terms of what you are able to do, and you will be able to develop a patience and tolerance with your body and heart, putting its needs first, which will help you to keep in good health constantly. Keep up the practice of pulse-taking as you move into different kinds of exercise – walking, exercises, and later swimming, cycling and climbing.

HOW TO TAKE YOUR OWN PULSE

METHOD I. Put two of your three middle fingers from either hand on the base of the thumb of the other hand, its palm outstretched. Slide the fingers an inch up the arm and feel the ridges of the two sharp bones which go to the elbow. Practise this for a while and feel into the hollow between the bones. Here you will find the pulse, and it is made easier to feel by pressing the pulse spot against the bone. If you can call upon the help of a nurse or friend who can show you how to take your pulse, this will be easier.

METHOD II. Stand with your back to the wall and look into a mirror. Raise one arm with the elbow bent and your hand with the palm facing your chest, so that your lower arm is vertical and the elbow pointing out. Place two of your fingers, index and the next one, onto your neck on the same side as your raised arm, parallel with your Adam's apple. Again, press the pulse against the bone to feel it stronger. You will need to practise this several times.

You will know from activities in the hospital how much exercise you have been able to take so far. Obviously the idea is not to overtax the system before it is properly repaired. Graduated exercises are best. Fifty paces one day, sixty the next, ten stairs first, or five, eventually walking to the post office or the pub. But there are no rules, and you can only judge what is best by your reaction to exercise. In the early days, the best guideline is isotonic exercises and NOT isometric, as shown in the table opposite.

ISOMETRIC	ISOTONIC
Weight lifting	Walking
Water skiing	Jogging
Horseback riding	Running
Decorating	Tennis
Furniture moving	Swimming
	Cycling
	Dancing

Obviously it is not good to get breathless or go blueish or bring on pain. If this occurs you have already done too much. You must stop *before* any of these symptoms occur. Little and often is the best prescription. Many people like a structure and like to work towards a goal, and setting reasonable goals is a good idea and good for morale. But the goals *must* be realistic. There is a danger of pushing yourself too far physically because you feel tired and have to exert yourself physically to compensate. If you can work towards walking to the pub for a pint on Sunday when you have come out of hospital two weeks previously, or to the park to sit under a tree, the achievement, if it is based on realism, will be spectacular. There is a fine balance here between having just enough motivation to get moving and get better, and getting into an overdrive pattern which is unhealthy.

Refer to the four personality types and work out from this which is the best way for you to get involved with exercise. Pretty well all four types will respond to the logic, structure and focus of some exercise programme, however modest. If you are of the intuitive type, you might want to take on more than you should in an attempt to get in touch with the bodily functions which have let you down in such an outrageous way. The physical type might try and become too competitive, especially if you join a gymnasium (which you will be very attracted to), where there are other people working out. There are now some very good gymnasiums that have a programme especially for the rehabilitation of coronary patients. Find out from your cardiologist or doctor what kind of structured exercise prog-ramme, organised under the control of a professional, is available in your area. If you are of the thinking type and are able to put your mind to it, you will appreciate the value of exercise and not deem it a waste of time, especially when you see the results. Exercise might be a more difficult task for the feeling type, as you may become moody when things don't work out as planned and stop half-way. You need some emotional support and you may need to share some activity with a friend or someone close and make it more fun. Most people, unless they are dedicated athletes, have difficulty keeping to an exercise programme and find their enthusiasm wanes after a week or so. It is important that some daily exercise becomes a habit – like cleaning your teeth. Something you don't think about or analyse too much.

In the early days after a heart attack you have the opportunity of establishing habits which can, in the future, offer you a lifeline, and I believe finding a kind of exercise that suits you is one of the most important of these lifelines. There is no medical evidence to prove that exercise prevents coronary artery disease or that it opens up arteries that have been narrowed by arteriole disease, but there is evidence that regular exercise contributes to the psychological wellbeing, to keeping physically fit and to keeping weight down by increasing the metabolic rate of the body.

One of the most important qualities about regular exercise is the disciplined ritual. If, at the end of the working day when perhaps you are tired, mentally or emotionally, perhaps rather bored, but unstretched physically, it is easy to just flop. You can then find that your tiredness becomes accentuated, that you feel even more sluggish and overcome with the events of the day and you may reach out to food and alcohol to 'perk' you up. If, on the other hand, you have organised a daily swim or run, or you have a mile walk from the station or a tennis game arranged, you may groan at the thought of exerting yourself, but once you are involved in physical exertion, that develops its own kind of momentum, banishing thoughts, sluggishness and a tendency to overthinking and depressive thinking. And afterwards the reward is a greater sense of wellbeing, of being in touch with your body; an all over physical sensation of functioning well and more energy rather than less to enjoy an evening.

Exercise has proved to be a lifeline for many people I know and have counselled during a difficult period. One woman I know feels that her daily track running kept her together after the tragic death of her husband. She had an appointment every morning and she faithfully kept it and it rewarded her with the realisation that if she could run every day, keep going when many of her instincts were to lie in bed and wait for something to happen, she was going to be able to look after herself. She got to like the bit of herself that said "come on, you can do it, this is important, this is one for you, this is your body, keep it as well-oiled as the engine of your car". Once again, it is important to distinguish between cardiac fatigue, brought on by overwork and exhaustion, and the everyday boredom and sluggishness that is lifted by exercise.

WALKING is the easiest and simplest exercise for starters. It can also relieve tension because it burns up energy as well as giving the walker something to do. There were many nights when my husband and I walked the streets of London because he came home tense, up-tight, unable to relax, on edge, after going back to work. In his book *Coronary Case*, Rex Edwards describes how several times after his coronary he felt such an overwhelming feeling of tension, of going to burst, or terror and fear, that he just had to get out and away and walk or drive until the feeling had passed. These feelings do need to be tackled at two levels, both emotionally and with a physical outlet for this pent-up energy force. See if you can make room for more walking.

You may find at first that pottering in the garden, going to collect your newspaper or taking the dog out form a routine for you.

When about three months has passed, ask your doctor if you might begin a more strenuous exercise programme. Some people will have sports or physical activity they are particularly fond of and after three months is the time to consider renewing them . . . perhaps you enjoy sailing, golf, tennis or squash. If you have not had much to do with sport, you might like to think about taking up something, particularly when you return to work or your previous routine. As I said earlier, this is a great time for making new beneficial habits and an excellent way of relieving tension and keeping the body fit and the circulation efficient.

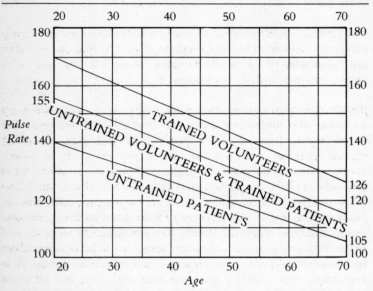

The British Pilot Study of exercise therapy examined the physiological and biochemical effects of a carefully graduated course of vigorous gymnasium training with two or three exercise sessions lasting only 15 minutes, in middle-aged London businessmen. Post-infarction patients underwent at least two months pre-treatment during which patients learnt to avoid overstrained states, control of anger-provoking situations and situations which provoked cardiac pain. They learnt about the effects of emotional stress and fatigue on cardiac performance; they met other people who had undergone the exercise programme and finally began the programme itself. A programme of graduated exercises, starting with basic simple stretching and mobilising exercises, which did not at any time exceed the prescribed heart rate and did not create sensations of more than moderate effort, developed week by week. Each person became able to accomplish the programme with slower pulse rates and greater ease. The above chart gives the pulse rate ranges for patients with cardiovascular disease at different stages of gymnasium training and is a useful guide to those beginning exercise without the facilities of a trained exercise therapist.

SWIMMING is ideal exercise if you are near a pool or are hardy enough to take on the nearest sea coast. In swimming the whole body is supported by water at the same time as being thoroughly exercised. Ten minutes a day or ten laps a day or three times each week is enough to keep fit.

CYCLING. This is excellent if you live in the country and many people cycle even in large cities these days. Cycling can be fitted into your way of life if you are able to use it as transport and once again the body is supported.

JOGGING is more strenuous, your body is not supported by anything else and more energy is demanded from you. It's worth trying because it's a quick, easy and cheap form of regular exercise and you can do it anywhere. It is worth investing in a good book on jogging if you are going to do it seriously. (There are some listed at the end of this book.) The main rule is to start slowly, 50 paces of jogging and then 50 paces of walking, repeated three or four times each day for one week, and then increased slowly to 75 paces and then 100, and so on. It is best to see how you feel about it and how your calves and ankles hold up after about a month. Once again, it is something you can do for ten minutes each day, and all of us can find ten minutes.

DANCING can be fantastic and many towns now have some kind of dance classes: modern, contemporary jazz, keep fit. If you like to exercise to music, and it does often make it more fun and less focused upon the exercise itself, joining a class would make lots of sense.

In his book *Aerobics*, Dr. Kenneth Cooper defines exercise in two parts . . . aerobic exercise is exercise which is sustained at a steady, vigorous level for a considerable period of time (more than ten minutes). This, he believes, develops endurance by elevating the heart rate and by its sustained use of oxygen strengthens the heart, lungs, blood vessels and other vital organs. Aerobics isn't one particular form of exercise, but the way in which it is carried out and one can exercise aerobically going upstairs or walking to work. The test is the sustained high pulse rate for over ten minutes, the feeling that you are being pushed and working hard, and the ability to be able to carry on a conversation, however staccato, with a companion.

When exercise is anaerobic it is either too slow to be effective unless sustained over a long period, or too strenuous, therefore causing 'oxygen debt' and exhaustion. The latter is an important point for people beginning an exercise programme. So many people do begin exercising in a rush, thinking they know how to do it and that they don't need any instruction; or they feel guilty that they don't exercise enough and rush to make up for lost time, or they forget their age, remembering, perhaps, the last time they exercised at school and presuming the same youth and vigour. It is indeed frightening what a sedentary life does to one's body and it's no good thinking that we will be able to run when we have to, or pick up where we left off years ago. We have all heard stories about the person who, on reading a magazine article in favour of exercise, suddenly decides to play an intense game of either squash or tennis, and, unfit and panting, he overstretches his physical capacity which either incapacitates him completely or puts him off trying exercise ever again.

If you are someone who has always exercised regularly, get back to it gradually. This may be hard at first, especially if you have been used to your body being flexible and reliable. Many people find they have to start almost from the beginning with their exercising after a heart attack but that after a few times of frustration and difficulty they quickly form their exercise habit again and maintain it without any trouble. The gym, or the place where you take your first strenuous steps back to exercising, may well become the place you recover your determination, morale, peace of mind and self-respect, as well as your body fitness. Exercise definitely carries with it many emotional feelings . . . those of wellbeing, of being in charge of oneself, and of the self-respect which comes when a hard battle, such as finding one's body strengths after serious illness, is won.

EFFORT

The heart's main function is to provide for the body's efforts. Many of us tend to think of effort as being physical ... that we are not really using our body unless we are running, walking or carrying something, and we can physically register the increased beats of our heart. But other kinds of activity affect the heart too, taking a more indirect route. *Remember that the heart is subordinate to the brain.* Coping with a busy schedule, whether it is within the home, office or on the road, where there are deadlines to meet, difficult people to deal with, unexpected problems and emotions with strangers or people we know, and having to cope with several different things at once, all take a toll on our thinking and feeling function, on our body as a whole and demand work from the heart. Many of us lead urban lives or live in inner cities and our daily routine involves travel of one sort or another which is becoming increasingly taxing and tiring. If we live in a run-down area, a high-rise flat, if we have a neglectful landlord, noisy neighbours or live with the constant fear of sudden violence, we have to make more effort than someone without these pressures.

One of the most important areas of effort which tends to get taken for granted is our dealings with other people and how these affect us. Talking to people, coping with their moods and demands can take a lot out of us. Dr. Peter Nixon uses the expression 'people poisoning' to describe the situation in which people become saturated with each other and each other's exchanges. We don't often stop to think about how people are affecting us, we just feel cross or defeated inside and shrug our shoulders, feeling we have no choice but to put up with things – or we find ourselves avoiding people or having sudden outbursts of anger and rage. Another factor which demands effort is an internal one – how much we feel inside ourselves that we can cope with the day's tasks ahead of us. Having to overcome internal feelings of defeat, hopelessness and helplessness when tasks seem to be too much all require a tremendous amount of effort before we can get started on the job in hand.

A useful way to find out how much effort your daily life requires is to make a map of all the different roles or 'people' you are in one day, and all the skills you have to use, all the emotions you are likely to engage in. For example a man might be:

(a) unsuccessful weightwatcher struggling with two extra stones
(b) father of three teenagers
(c) gardener at weekends for 1½ acres
(d) fast car driver
(e) debtor to building society, bank
(f) responsible for annual accounts and budget
(g) reluctant patient resenting waste of time
(h) employer of two workers for small-mail order business at home
(i) head of local golf club
(j) manager of fourteen men at work
(k) husband
(l) governor of son's school
(m) son of widowed mother with frequent angina

(Taken from 'Once Individuals Can Recognise Stress, Counselling Can Help' E. Wilde McCormick, *General Practitioner Magazine*, 1984)

Each of these areas has a whole variety of expression, and some days we have to attend in detail to more than three or four areas. When you break down the kind of life you are leading and roles you are playing into sections like this, you can get a clear idea of how much you are asking of yourself. Learning how to map out our weeks and our days by taking into consideration everything that we ask ourselves and working towards a realistic balance is the way that we stay healthy and working well. A sign of getting out of balance is when we find ourselves trying to cram another entire job into the half hour we have to 'spare' between a dental appointment and our next customer. Much better to use the time for relaxation and pleasure. Finding time – five minutes, half an hour throughout the day to top up our energy bank can be a life saver – and is certainly an energy saver. It is much better to keep topping up your reserves than it is to ask the body to go steamrollering ahead without a break so that you can 'get it all over with'. Experience tells us that this never works ... we never really feel finished, we are often too exhausted at going flat out to enjoy ourselves when we do stop, and our 'having to' wait to enjoy ourselves until every single 'i' is dotted encourages us to be compulsive in our behaviour which spills over into other areas in our life. Remember, everything that you do is asking the heart for more effort, more blood to the muscles, more oxygen to cope with fatigue and so raised pulse and raised blood pressure. When we overload ourselves continually our body's natural self-regulatory process cannot stand up to the onslaught and we begin a pattern of ill-health.

The heart patient needs all fitness and stamina he can get. He also needs to know and understand his limits, to say no, to stop when appropriate and that he has good days and bad days. When you have made your individual map of rules, look at how much preparation you have had for fulfilling these notes, whether any are redundant or could be delegated or shared. See what the gaps are that need to be attended to so that you may be freed from unnecessary anxiety and pressure.

b. Sex

Although sex is freely talked about in the media and by young people, many older people find it difficult to talk about, and many people who are married feel that they should be able to sort these things out for themselves and not need any consultation. But after a serious illness the resumption of sexual activity is extremely important for health, for release of tension and, perhaps most important, for the assertion identity and confidence.

For a man, the fear of not being able to make love after a heart attack, of being impotent, being unable to sustain an erection, and fear of having another heart attack or even dying whilst making love, can be at the root of sexual difficulties after a serious illness, and can put couples off even attempting to resume their sexual life together. If the fear remains, is not aired or discussed, it can grow out of proportion. Sadly too, many people do not enjoy a happy and fulfilling sexual life and these problems are likely to be exaggerated after a heart attack, or the attack is used as an excuse for not bothering to have any sexual activity at all. On the other hand, a heart attack gives both you and your partner an ideal opportunity to 'start again' with your sexual life, in finding out what pleases each of you, and because you have to go slowly, to take one experience at a time.

What we come to know about sex is a miscellaneous collection of information learned in fragmented pieces, picked up from contemporaries, overheard from 'experts', seen in magazines, shown in films at school when we were younger. All this external information is a long way removed from what happens to the way we relate it to ourselves and our own experience. Even with all the information available today it is quite possible for someone to grow up not fully realising the implications of such information for him or herself, and in no way able to relate what he or she has learned to their own bodies. I well remember being shown a film about menstruation when I was twelve and in a local high school but I really didn't think it would ever happen to me. Many of us, now in our late thirties, forties or fifties, grew up with these kinds of experiences and the way our sex lives have been formulated has been a hotchpotch of different kinds of stimuli. At the same time, we have witnessed the birth of an incredible openness about sex and sexual habits. The apparent freedom which young people enjoy today may well be something that did not occur in our youth. The freedom to talk about sexual problems and feelings may never have been one you have claimed.

Before looking at ways in which we may build a satisfactory sexual life with a partner whom we love, we will have to take a look at many of the responses that have possibly become a habit, taken for granted. This is a time when you can begin to say and discover what you like to do to each other because now you have the wonderful permission of time to let you explore. Because the heart attack has changed the way in which everything happens at first, let it have this effect on your sex life.

Some hospitals do give advice about resuming sexual life and some do not. It is important to ask and to discuss this with your doctor if you can. It is best not to focus on the act of intercourse, about 'when' it is going to happen. The most important thing you can do after someone has had a heart attack, has survived and has returned home, is to hold and hug them a lot. Many people feel a sense of violation after serious illness or surgery, as if their body has been invaded, and they may feel fragile and wounded, not just actually physically but emotionally and psychologically. Touch has a restorative and healing quality, especially when it comes from someone you love or care deeply about. Later, when you feel like sharing some more intimate stroking and cuddling, you can feel your body gradually waking up again. It can be very good to feel this way and important too that it doesn't have to 'lead' to anything else. I met several women who were afraid to enjoy this kind of intimate playing in case it leads to their husbands getting aroused sexually and putting the heart under stress. One woman I met had moved herself out of the bedroom to sleep on a camp bed because of this fear! Very few people have a heart attack whilst making love. In his study on the so-called co-ition death, Ueno found that only 0.6% of 5,559 cases of sudden death were precipitated by sexual activity and three-quarters of these were associated with extramarital intercourse. Your doctor may have given you a guideline as to when to start having intercourse again – when you can climb two flights of stairs without pain of breathlessness, perhaps four to five weeks after your heart attack. But the best guideline is your pulse level. When you can safely allow your pulse to get to 120 (this needs to be discussed with your doctor) you can have intercourse, which does raise the pulse considerably and puts up the blood pressure. Of course, there will be concern about performance at first, and until you feel physically fit again, this will affect what happens. If you can remove anxiety, fear of not performing as you feel you 'ought' and hurry, you will find that your body will gradually show you, and your partner, what it most needs sexually and sensually as each day changes.

My feeling about sex is that it has somehow become such a competitive, misunderstood, chauvinistic (on both sides) subject and has got far too far removed from the human relationship within which it is naturally embedded. Sex is the friendliest of the sharing experiences, one of the most pleasurable, quite the most accepting of all the combinations of human endeavour. It is within the sexual framework that we build respect, learn acceptance and begin to value both ourselves and the other person for what they are at the core. Whenever there is a problem with sex in a partnership it is often related to the trust and confidence that the particular relationship holds.

When the individual thinks only of his or her own pleasure, or judges the other's performance by something read in magazines or reported by other people, there is no hope for any fun or any pleasure. So often when sex is wrong in a relationship the rest of the relationship founders from this point, or it causes such irritation and lack of respect that other areas that might have had the potential for success and togetherness fail because what is at deepest source is off-centre.

If you have never had a good sex life together, or if there has always been something that bothered you about it, niggled away, made you puzzled, the crisis of illness is the ideal time to get all these things sorted out. Do a lot of homework on your own. Read books, read articles and magazines, digest the ones that are helpful in terms of meaning something to you in your own life and your own reality. Discard what your common sense tells you is irrelevant or not your scene or cup of tea. But investigate . . . look at the book list at the end of this book. If you have already been thinking about who it is you've been living with all these years, ponder on this aspect of them. You know what pleases them . . . or do you? Do you know what pleases you? Do you feel guilty or naughty about thinking about these things . . . do you think somehow they're bad . . . that sex should just work out in a relationship, like making the tea in the mornings? Well, in that you are wrong. Sex, although the most instinctual and natural of our functions is actually quite difficult. It doesn't 'just happen'. What was once instinctual is now wrapped up with sociological ideals, pressure from Society and the family, pressures from the Church and our culture. All of us experience an ambivalent attitude towards sex as we grow up and try to attain a sexual identity for ourselves. We know the feelings that we have in our bodies and that seem so natural, but, at the same time, so often we are told that they are bad, we shouldn't have them and therefore we are bad. Or we are told that we have to fight against the sins of the flesh and the temptation of the Devil. Society's attitude to sex has been to 'black' a person because of his sexual preferences . . . look at the way we talk about homosexuals, as though their entire personality was governed by their sexual choice. It is difficult to throw off a lifetime of sexual opinions and social mores and it can't be done overnight, but this time is a good time to try and begin.

We have talked about sex so far as something we share with partners, male or female. What happens if we have no sexual partner? It does not follow that because one has a partner one is sexy and if there is no-one around one is not. We remain sexual beings whoever is around and our appetite is totally individual. Some people can have long periods of celibacy and be quite happy about it. I have found that people do use their creative libido, or sexual energy, in different ways such as intense religious or other profound experience, extreme periods of hard work, during the production of a 'great work'. Their libido or life force has become directed and focused onto something else, and often fantastic creative achievements are born. Also, during a family crisis or illness, and the later stages of pregnancy, people have less sexual energy, especially if they are under stress. I believe that when we make a conscious choice about the use of our sexual energy, this channelling is appropriate and healthy, and the periods of time involved, however long, always come to an end. What is less healthy is avoidance, putting off, getting into lazy habits or not facing one's immediate situation fully. This does happen when we are depressed or under great stress.

If you have no sexual partner and long for the relief of orgasm this can be found through masturbation. It is not wrong and will not make you mad or blind. It is something that you can give to yourself as a gift; you may like to think of it as something you give yourself as a source of energy because it relieves the tension that builds up when sexual energy has found no expression. Or you may like to think of it as merely a necessary temporary measure, an emergency need. Many people do carry on masturbating even when they have a sexual partner because their needs are greater than the other's, and this does not indicate any perversion, as I have heard suggested. Of course masturbation will not make up for not having a relationship and the warmth of another person, and people have told me that it accentuates their loneliness. This must be a personal decision. Masturbation is not wrong; it brings about a profound psychological expression which is extremely beneficial and healthy and we all face loneliness at some time or another. If loneliness is an important underlying issue in your life and has been for some time, the reasons for it need to be examined thoroughly and some alleviation sought. I refer to this again in Section k.

Perhaps you are thinking that at your age you should be past enjoying sex, or that maybe in a few years you won't have to think about it any more, or that you wish you didn't have to bother about it, or that at least with this illness it will give an excuse to give it a miss? If you have any of these thoughts, please think again. Very, very hard. By denying the pleasure of sex and the intimacy that is enclosed within it you are denying both you and your partner the possibility of experiencing the greatest physical pleasures man and woman have available to them; you are denying yourselves closeness, and you are denying your partner a healthy future. Sexual satisfaction is a vitally important part of the recovery from illness. It restores warmth and intimacy, it restores respect, it restores feeling of hope, it restores those intimate gender feelings of being a man or being a woman . . . what other experience is there in which you can truly say how much you feel like a man or like a woman? Physiologically it exercises the body and the circulation and works the lungs, but far more profound is the sense of exhilaration of being alive as a sexual being. And here I'm not talking about performance of any kind . . . there really is no criteria for good or bad sex, and at the time following illness the emphasis should be on reviving the sensual pleasures such as holding, caressing, stroking, licking, kissing, touching, cuddling, nuzzling, smiling, looking, watching . . . bathing together, sitting naked together . . . just these kind of things.

To excite the sensuality within each of you without the threat of having to (or not) make the big time at the end is the most important use of your private time together . . . these times may last for days, weeks or months. It will also give you a chance to see how your pulse rate responds to these kinds of stimuli, to watch how you feel, to learn to trust your body to allow pleasure again after it has given you so much pain. So often anxiety about performance gets in the way of simply having a playful time; well, after illness you have the excuse, or permission, to play like children, discovering each other's bodies, each other's pleasures, making each other feel acceptable, good and loved. All this may lead finally to intercourse. Sometimes it's best to try for the first few times with the woman on top, or lying on your side. A little gentle oral sex may be acceptable for both of you, and all the time you are loving each other, building confidence, trust and admiration.

A satisfactory, rich and full sex life is one of the surest ways to health. In being able to express our sexual needs we are also expressing something of what we feel is our basic value, and we are asking for that value to be confirmed by another on its most intimate level. In interviews with heart attack patients the fact of repressed sexuality emerged on many occasions . . . there is something in the fact that the denial of the 'heart' feelings . . . those romantic, personal intimate qualities within man that are expressed within a sexual relationship, can be 'blocked', or cause a blockage under which the heart protests, as by the example of illness. This is something we will discuss further in Chapter 7.

c. Food, Eating and Diet

Every magazine we pick up these days contains an article about the hazards or joys of certain foods: food allergies, cholesterol, fibre, about salt and chemicals, about preservatives, about foods which make us fat, diets which make us fat or offer a miracle cure to overweight, and about foods which are 'bad' and foods which are 'good'. Everyone has their special miracle diet or idea about food and diet, an idea which they claim can change your life.

One thing is very sure and that is that eating habits formed after a lifetime cannot be changed overnight. In fact I would say that changing your diet is one of the hardest adjustments to make during recovery. The first thing to look at is whether you need to change your eating habits. Because there are so many different views of food it can be very confusing to ascertain whether your own diet is healthy or not. But here are some broad basic facts and some suggestions. Can you answer "yes" to any of the following:

1   Do you eat a large number of fried meals, especially meals fried in lard or meals comprised of fried fatty meats such as pork or breast of lamb? (A large number would range from five times per week on the low scale to one or more fatty meals every day)
2   Are many of your meals tinned, processed, frozen or convenience (take away) foods? (Again, five meals a week to one every day)
3   Do you add salt to every meal?
4   Are you more than 10lbs overweight?
5   Do you have high blood pressure or suffer from oedema (fluid retention)?
6   Do you suffer from arthritis, sinusitis, gout, hayfever?
7   Do you often get constipated?

If you can answer "yes" to any of these then you do need to consider a change in your diet. This will help you not just with your heart condition but also with your weight, your general fitness, energy level and sense of wellbeing. We are, after all, what we eat, and the fact of so many different, albeit confusing reports on food values does indicate Society's general awareness of the need to find a healthy diet. Altering a lifetime of dietary habits cannot be achieved instantly. We are talking here of long-established patterns that go back to before our births . . . what our mother ate when she was nursing us, what food was available when we were growing up and the family's attitude to food, eating, and to mealtimes.

Let's start by examining our priorities and our food habits. Are we interested in food or do we just make it as easy and simple as possible and get it over with as quickly as possible? Do we have a weight problem or have to be on a special diet because of diabetes, ulcers, hypertension or anything else? Or do we love food very much, enjoying shopping for food and preparing it? Are mealtimes something special for us? Is food a problem, do we worry about it, about cooking it? Do we have only a vague idea about nutrition, about food values, food additives which are harmful, do we only 'know' a limited selection of foods? Now that you are involved in the convalescence business what you eat and how you eat will bring food much more into consciousness for you. Whatever your previous habits and whatever your answers to the above set of questions, it will be important to check on what you are eating. Food forms two main functions: to keep us alive and to act as a form around which we communicate socially.

In our house, mealtimes offer the one focal point at which we all get together, however we are all getting on and whatever the problems we might be suffering from. They are therefore extremely important. Three or four times each week, during school time and holidays, we all sit down together to a meal which several of us have helped to prepare in one way or another. It has a ritualistic effect. We light candles, take trouble over the presentation, sometimes having flowers and proper napkins, separate dishes for serving, depending on how much time we have had that day; or we might have just a simple meal like wholemeal bread and salad, or one dish of pasta, but the occasion will have the same feeling as if we had laid on a feast. My personal view is that meals are the centre of family life, whatever the size of the family; that they are to be lingered over in the evenings as much as possible and not organised around television programmes. Also, if you are the one in charge of cooking and shopping you have an ideal opportunity to see that everyone in your family gets a reasonably balanced diet. It takes effort and many people I know complain about the effort involved but it's worth it in terms of health and it pays off in terms of communication. Both these points are an essential part of convalescence and the time is there to put more into organising what you eat and how you eat it.

My priorities, then, are taste, food value, presentation and communication, in that order. I suggest you make a list of the foods you eat normally in one week; get each member of your family to do his or her own list as people often eat differently in the same family. Then ask each one to make another list of meals they would have liked to have, or have more of, and ones which seem to crop up too often and have become boring or tasteless. I do think that people's food interests change, come in phases, and that these changes often coincide with other changes that are going on in our lives; often with climate, time of the year, outside interests, taste buds. One wonderful thing that does begin to happen when we think seriously about food and start asking our taste buds to make decisions for us is that our palate becomes much more sensitive and refined, much more discerning, and it is our palate with which we should work most.

Having had a look at what our eating habits are and what sort of foods we like, the second task is to weed out the foods which are not doing us any good and change the emphasis on certain foods if it appears that we are eating too much of one thing.

Let's look at some of the subjects that are most written about today.

ANIMAL FAT

The recent cholesterol theory proves statistically that there is a strong relationship between the intake of saturated fat (animal fats), high blood fats (especially cholesterol) and coronary artery disease. This theory has recently been disputed in medical circles (see section on Cholesterol under title *"Who has a Heart Attack?"*) but there are other reasons why cutting down on the amount of animal fat in our diet is beneficial. This is to do with the toxins and acidity that are built up in the bloodstream by a diet high in animal fat, and which affect our circulation, endocrine gland efficiency, the flexibility of our joints, and our mucous membrane secretions. Cutting out dairy products alone can relieve symptoms of sinusitis, hayfever and arthritis, and I have seen many examples of success in this area. Even if you did not have a high blood cholesterol level during your hospital tests it is not a bad idea to cut down on animal fat and dairy products. Also, a diet high in fat is high in calories and this inclines us to overweight, another risk factor in coronary artery disease. Switching to sunflower seed oil, safflower oil, olive or any *vegetable* oil, rather than using lard or any of the hard cooking fats; using polyunsaturated fat such as *Flora* rather than butter; grilling any meat or bacon that you eat rather than frying it, using a non-stick pan or Chinese wok to 'pan fry' foods which are only lightly oiled with a pastry brush or are not oiled at all; all these will help. It really is surprising how easily one can become adjusted to eating less fat. The easiest way is not to buy fatty meats like pork or breast of lamb but to buy, perhaps more expensive, but leaner, cuts of meat much less often, say, once or twice a week, instead of every day. This does mean changing perhaps lifetime habits of meat and two vegetables, and it would only seem to be necessary if you see from your week's food intake that you do, indeed, eat 6oz or more of fatty meats per day, and particularly if you see that you eat more than five meals a week which have been fried. Cutting down on fatty meat and frying using polyunsaturated fat and vegetable oil is the easiest way to reduce the fats we eat. But it's important to remember that fats are also present in a 'hidden' way in biscuits, cakes, pastries, sauces, gravy, puddings, oily fish and, of course, all dairy products are high in fat content. Once again, if you find you are eating a large number of cakes or biscuits which contain a lot of fat, try eating them every other day instead of every day, or just at weekends instead of several times a week. Eat eggs two or three times a week, and if you are a great cheese consumer, try some of the low or medium fat cheeses like curd cheeses, Edam and Gouda cheese, cottage cheese or some types of Brie. Some nutritionists advise cutting out all cheeses altogether and this may be something you decide to do, but remember that changes need to be approached gradually.

FIBRE

There is now overwhelming evidence that Western countries

have made themselves more prone to a whole series of diseases – diabetes, bowel disorders and possibly heart disease, by a diet too high in fat, refined sugars and carbohydrates and too low in natural fibre. The Third World countries, whose diet is primarily fibre from vegetables and grain, do not suffer from these diseases in quantity. The diet factor has been isolated from this research. Dietary fibre is obtained from plants as opposed to animals. Generally, foods high in fibre, such as nuts, breakfast cereals and wholewheat pasta, require more chewing, tend to provide more bulk in the stomach and the feeling of satisfaction after eating is longer lived. Sometimes people say about fibre-high foods "that won't fill me up" or "that won't give me much nourishment", but this is, in fact, an unfortunate myth which must have grown from the days in which protein was thought to be the main source of food value. Two ounces of brazil nuts give as much protein as a steak, but with more vitamins and a high amount of fibre. Baked beans on wholemeal toast serves an easy, tasty, highly nutritious meal; wholemeal pasta served with a sauce made with tomatoes and tunafish is delicious, high in vitamins, fibre and enough protein to last us a whole day.

OVERWEIGHT

If you are overweight by more than 10% you should seriously think about choosing a diet which will reduce this load you are carrying. Being overweight is one of the main risk factors in heart disease and in being overweight you run the risk of other diseases. Disorders involving the circulation and joints, diabetes and high blood pressure can be greatly improved by weight loss in an overweight person.

If you are overweight and have been so for a number of years have a look at your eating and living habits, at some of the reasons why you eat more than you need. Often being overweight is because we have bad habits; we eat too much of the 'wrong' foods and we sit about a lot and this pattern forms a vicious circle. We have two polarities working in this country, that of great emphasis on being slim and slimming programmes and foods; and the vast selection of food we have to choose from, especially frozen pre-prepared meals, easy take-away meals and the largest confectionery selection and consumption in the world.

How very difficult, then, for someone who has a poor relationship with food, who does not know when to stop eating or how to regulate eating appropriately, who uses food as a comfort, a friend, an escape, to know where to place himself sensibly, and how easy it is for him to swing from one extreme to another, dieting one week, over-eating the next. This is extremely bad for us. There are many, many diets and diet books and magazines. Ask your doctor to give you a diet, or choose a low-fat, high fibre diet from one of the books in your local bookshop and stick to it as hard as you can. The focus is that you are changing your eating habits in order to live more happily and healthily, and it's important to focus on this rather than on a feeling of being deprived.

There are some things you can do in preparation for dieting. One is to have a look at your eating habits honestly, laying them down on paper and facing honestly just how much you are eating without realising – those often forgotten snacks like chocolate bars on the train and the packet of crisps before supper. Another is to ask yourself what you need your fat for . . . is it to give you more space in the world where you are afraid to ask? Is it to give you ballast, to hold you down and stop you flying off somewhere with your ideas; is it to make you feel closer to the earth, to ground you when you are unbounded; is it to hide the true shape of your body, to hide your sexuality so that you don't have to do anything about it? Now that serious illness has erupted into your life, are you ready to give it up . . . in fact, can you afford to hide behind your fat or lug it around with you? Dieting is much easier when you have decided that you can do without extra body fat and you are ready psychologically to shed weight. As the process of weight loss goes on you may be more aware of your vulnerability to certain things – to being sexual, for example, if this is what your weight was hiding. When we begin to confront the things we have been afraid of and have therefore been hiding from we do feel exposed at first and this is when it is tempting to rush back into old patterns. If you have made conscious what it is you are shielding within yourself and have been able to put it in its appropriate context, this process is much easier to go through. If you need more space, your task is to learn to be assertive enough to ask for it rather than putting food into your body to make it large enough to do it for you.

Choose a diet which suits your lifestyle and your taste buds and try and make the food you eat as interesting as possible. It is important to lose weight slowly and that you replace an unsatisfactory eating habit with a healthier one, for life. It is important, too, not to make this task too arduous at this particular time as this period of recovery is hard enough without adding unnecessary strain. It helps if one or more members of your family joins you in your new eating way, that you do not sit separate with your calorie counted platter. It is easy enough for the person cooking to make one dish suitable for everyone and let those who are not slimming have something extra in addition to the person losing weight rather than a completely separate menu. There are some extremely good diet books on the market with pictures and menus exciting enough for any group to enjoy together.

JUNK FOOD

Junk food is primarily food which goes bland as soon as you put it in your mouth. It may look good and smell good, but it soon converts to a tasteless mass in your mouth and a heavy lump in your stomach. How often have you been desperate enough to eat a stodgy pork pie or Cornish pastie full of gristle and potato, or a fatty hamburger with violently coloured gherkin and ketchup which leaves a red stain on your tongue, only to have it turn into a tasteless, hopeless pulp? It is also usually high in fat, salt, sugar, preservatives and colouring. It is a bit of a trap and all too often a big disappointment. Once in a while this might be fun, but it is certainly not advisable to get into the habit of eating such rubbish. It pays, therefore, to be selective about what junk food you do eat, if at all. Some hamburgers are, in fact, delicious, well prepared with salad in a wholemeal bun and have a fair proportion of food values. There are several calorie guides to junk foods. Have a look at what you are putting into your system before you allow yourself to be swayed by hunger and the temptation of the moment.

POTASSIUM

Diets high in potassium are recommended for patients taking diuretic drugs such as thiazides and drugs such as digitalis and the other anti-arrhythmic drugs. These drugs can cause the loss of potassium from the myocardial cells. When there is a deficiency in potassium in the body muscular weakness is experienced, abnormal heart rhythms, lethargy, kidney and lung deficiencies and failure. The main rôles of potassium are for muscle contraction, maintenance of fluid and electrolyte balance in cells, transmission of nerve impulses and the release of energy from carbohydrates, proteins and fats. No special supplement is needed but foods rich in potassium such as bananas, orange juice, dried fruits, unsalted nuts, peanut butter, dried beans and peas, bran and potatoes should be included in the diet to help balance the body's muscular and thermal energy, and high potassium diets are recommended for all post-coronary patients, whether they are on drugs or not.

SALT

After sugar, salt is the leading food additive. The actual amount required to keep the average body in good health is only one tenth of a teaspoonful a day, and this is found in its natural form in most foodstuffs without adding any salt whatsoever to our diet. Salt in the form of sodium is found in foods from the ground, and from animals, and it is in all preservatives. Too much salt encourages the retention of fluid in the body tissue and research shows that this is linked with high blood pressure. Salt, like alcohol, is a 'learned' taste, something that we get used to, that becomes a habit, and it is one which has to be broken gradually. In cutting down salt intake it is important to look also at the tinned or processed foods you are eating for the sodium content. There are 'hidden' amounts of salt in many breakfast cereals, in instant puddings, in canned soups, all packaged and frozen foods, high sodium vegetables such as sauerkraut, olives and pickles. When you begin to cut down on salt intake your palate will tell you which foods contain salt, and you will gradually not need or crave for salt to be added. As part of your programme to cut down on salt, experiment with using herbs and spices instead: lemon juice, chives, bay leaf, garlic – the list is endless.

CAFFEINE

Coffee and tea both contain caffeine. The average cup of tea (one spoonful of tea leaves) contains 41 milligrams of caffeine, about half that of brewed coffee and two-thirds that of instant coffee. Tea brewed from tea bags tends to have less caffeine than loose tea. Cola drinks also contain caffeine. Caffeine is absorbed immediately into the blood and stimulates the central nervous system. This produces an alert state (jitteriness if too much is drunk) and a more rapid heartbeat, triggers the release of insulin which causes our blood sugar to drop and makes us to feel hungry, and also acts as a diuretic.

There is no evidence that moderate caffeine intake (one or two cups of tea or coffee per day) increases the risk of heart disease, but large quantities can produce an abnormally fast heartbeat with an abnormal rhythm or extra beats. Coffee has been known to induce heartburn if drunk on an empty stomach. During the initial stages of convalescence it would be wise to cut down caffeine intake to a minimum, or not take any at all. Instead you could try herbal teas . . . mint, camomile or raspberry, or drink decaffeinated coffee, cocoa (made with skimmed milk) or simply hot water and lemon . . . an acquired taste, I know, but this can become a very refreshing drink with a cleansing after-effect once you get used to it.

Stopping a large coffee or tea habit takes time. Caffeine is addictive and you may find that you crave for it at first when you try and cut down. Remember that this will pass, it will get less and less bad and that by not giving in to it you are helping to lessen the next bout of craving. Try some of the non-addictive alternatives and, if your imagination will allow, pretend to yourself that your new drink has the same delicious properties of the one you have cut down on and that you are going to feel just as good!

SUGAR

Too much sugar causes overweight; once again, it has addictive properties and can, through overproduction of insulin, convert blood glucose into fatty acids and triclycerides. It is the latter which can promote the development of atherosclerosis. Sugar has no food value other than to create body fat. It is habit forming, causing us to have a sweet tooth so that we crave satisfaction from more sugar-loaded foodstuffs. Worst of all, there is no need for us to consume refined sugar at all. If we eat fresh fruit, vegetables and bread, we get all the natural sugar we need when this food is processed during digestion. Once again, sugar should be cut down gradually. Stop taking it in drinks first, then adding it to food, and cut down on sweet puddings. Look at the amount of sugar in some of the packaged foods you buy . . . cereals, for instance, and bread and cake. Make sure you eat only a limited amount . . . say, one sweet item every day . . . and that this forms a 'treat'.

DIETARY GOALS

So what do we end up eating after all this? "There's nothing much left", you may be groaning. Go back to the list you made of what you like to eat and match it with some of the things we have talked about here. Concentrate on the major areas . . . maybe you have been eating too many dairy products or too many sweets. Try cutting these down for starters and, at the same time, try one or two easier things . . . maybe you aren't that bothered about salt and can start cutting out without any difficulty. Maybe you have more time to prepare food and can enjoy experimenting with freshly cooked meals or with the vegetables from your garden. See what you personally can cope with best and gradually begin to make changes here and there.

A rough guide to the proportions of protein, carbohydrate and fat is to divide these into the following proportions . . . over half to be consumed as carbohydrate, mainly complex carbohydrates such as wholemeal bread or pasta or beans, vegetables, fruit and pulses with less than one-fifth simple carbohydrates like cakes and sugars; less than one-third of our diet to take the form of fats like polyunsaturated fat, skimmed milk, low fat cheeses, and the 'hidden' fats from lean meat, eggs, fish and about 12% to 15% of our diet to be taken in protein. Again, lean meat and fish, nuts, eggs, poultry, hard cheeses. You will see that the most up-to-date dietary information recommends much less protein every day than many of us think we need. The idea of protein being the main source of goodness in our diet seems to have grown with the affluence of the Western World. As people become more wealthy they tend to purchase more meat, butter and cheeses, perhaps believing that because these things were out of reach because of poverty or war, they were to be strived for and consumed in great quantities the minute hardships no longer applied. A rough guideline is six ounces of protein per day for a 150lb adult. Since all foods contain a mixture of protein, carbohydrate and fat, as well as water, what you are getting in your six ounces of protein is not pure protein but the amount in proportion which has been worked out as advisable for your needs. Since you may be getting much of your protein from vegetables, bread and fruit, it is best to limit your heavier protein to two x two ounce portions per day, or one x three ounce portion and one cheese portion. It is useful in going into these kinds of details to buy yourself a book giving the different food and calorie values for each food so that you can be more accurate.

If you are the one responsible for cooking and looking after a heart attack patient, I would recommend you spend at least one morning in a bookshop looking at cookery books based on sound nutritional ideas; that you pick one or two and you stick to them. There are books which cater especially for heart patients, and I have listed these in the book list at the end. You might enjoy these, but don't load yourself with too much which is too complicated, too soon. You want to go slowly, get yourself used to possibly new ways of buying and handling food, and as you are the cook you might have to entice your patient with new dishes that he might, at first, resent or be suspicious of. He might revert to childishness, demanding his nursery sustenance, and there is no harm in this at all. He has had a major illness and he will need some pandering to . . . it's a mistake to withdraw all the things he likes, however 'bad' they are made out in the health books; this will just make him moody and depressed and he won't enjoy his food at all, which is not the idea. So at first it's a balance . . . a slow re-education, if this is necessary, to better, healthier eating habits. And you have to be involved, too, for it's no use making him special meals and making him feel a freak, and yourself getting resentful because you have to work on two separate meals. It won't do you or your family any harm to eat more healthily, and the trick would be to include everyone in a choice of dishes. Spending an evening, perhaps, going over some of the recipes, finding out how much your family want to experiment. Often teenagers refuse to eat anything new and stare in hostility at something you've worked for hours to produce. It's just too bad. They will eat if they are hungry. But they, too, have had a shock and have to make an adjustment. Their noses may have been put out of joint by Dad's illness and they might be feeling uncertain and afraid. It's important for them to feel that things are basically the same at home and so too many changes in too extreme a way are not a good idea.

Don't feel you've failed if at first your desire to change the family's eating pattern doesn't appear to have succeeded. It won't work all at once, and it isn't your failure to make your partner give up his fried food, or whatever, that will make him ill again. Heart disease begins long before the onset of an attack. It is an accumulation of long term events and although you cannot change this, you can encourage a better and healthier attitude in your partner which he then has the responsibility to take on.

SOME DIETARY MYTHS

"Haphazard eating habits and too much instant or junk food can be compensated by handfuls of vitamin, mineral or trace element capsules." This is not so. Nutritious sweeteners such as honey and molasses have, in fact, no more beneficial value used in the quantities in which sugar is usually added. No health foods can 'cure' or prevent disease. They may help to provide us with a healthier diet and this may have a cumulative effect, but this is all.

'Natural' foods do not necessarily mean good foods. The potato, for example, contains 150 different chemicals. In her recent book on nutrition, Jane Brody writes: "If it were possible to eat your year's quota of potatoes – 120lbs all at once – you'd be killed outright by the 10,000 milligrams of solanine, a relative of the poison in deadly nightshade". The emphasis here is on quantity, and this is where it is important and valuable to vary your diet so that a build-up of chemicals is less likely to take place.

Here are some simple priorities which, in my view, could make that vitally important contribution to your changing to a healthier diet:

1 Eat less than you did before the heart attack, smaller portions at mealtimes and fewer, or at best no, snacks between meals.

2 Eat one main meal a day, preferably at lunchtime or 6.00pm. Food eaten late at night has less chance of being digested as efficiently or of being used up in energy than food eaten during the daytime.

3 Complement your one main meal with one or two smaller meals, balanced to provide your daily nutritional needs.

4 Eat small portions of saturated fat and aim to cut these down to three times per week, supplementing some of the alternative foods we've mentioned to give you protein and vitamins. Stop frying in deep saturated fats altogether . . . use pan-frying, steaming, grilling, cooking with herbs or lemon juice in the oven. If you have been 'addicted' to fried foods and eaten them all your life, cut down slowly, aiming

at only the occasional fried meal. The traditional fried meal can now be composed of oven chips, baked eggs, grilled bacon and sausages.

5   Revise your ideas about carbohydrate foods and include more fibre – vegetables, wholemeal bread, brown rice, wholemeal pasta, grains and pulses, into your diet.

6   No added salt or refined sugar.

7   Buy fresh food rather than tinned, processed, frozen or take-away foods.

8   Start growing your own herbs on your window sill in pots and get used to cutting off a few fresh shoots as you are cooking.

9   Concentrate on taste, quality, variety, moderation and savouring these four.

d.   Alcohol

If you like and enjoy the odd drink it will be good to know that alcohol, in moderation, can actually help you, especially during convalescence. There are some claims that alcohol drinkers have higher levels of high density lipoproteins in their blood which act as protective agents against the deposit of fatty substances in the arteries. Also, moderate consumption of alcohol can reduce stress and tension and help to relax tense muscles. However, it is moderation that must be stressed and by this we mean a maximum of one or two drinks per day, one whisky and a glass of wine and so on. Excess of alcohol will not improve matters, whereas in moderation it may well do so.

Too much alcohol can be devastating to your health and to your social life. Big consumers of alcohol are far more likely to raise their blood pressure, damage heart muscle, gain weight, eat poorly and live an irregular life, not exercising or sleeping properly, or die early from diabetes, stroke or heart disease than those who drink only in moderation. Alcohol is a toxic drug, toxic to the brain, heart, liver, kidneys and gastro-intestinal tract and to sexual performance in men and women. It is also a proven fact now that alcohol impairs performance. Recent tests by a medical group studying alcoholism showed that, after two pints of beer or one and a half gins, the work performance is impaired by eleven per cent. If you are struggling to do a job, any kind of job, what you do will be slower and less accurate after this amount of alcohol. Frustration develops when the output is less than personal satisfaction demands, and in terms of having had a coronary, this is not a happy state of affairs. In the evening, when you can sit down and enjoy a drink, these effects are not so crucial, and in this situation alcohol can offer you much. Remember to savour your one or two glasses each day. Save them for when you can really enjoy them and not gulp them down, sip them in a tranquil atmosphere. If you are on any medication, check with your doctor that alcohol will not impair the effect of the drugs you are on. Narcotics, tranquillisers, anti-depressants, antihistamines and sleeping pills become more potent when mixed with alcohol and should not come near each other.

If you have a drink problem and the heart attack has forced you to recognise it, discuss this with someone; either your doctor or a counsellor, and get some help with drawing up a plan for making changes. You will probably have to find out why you need to drink to excess, or how this need became a habit, and then work on a programme for breaking the habit. Often people drink to give themselves courage, to blot out pain, to kill time; sometimes when we can't bear to face something or we want to hide what we consider a weakness, we turn to the blanketing effects of alcohol and live in this limbo state, tricked by its apparent safety, like an ostrich with its head in the sand. But our bodies don't go on forever and our psyche directs us towards life events in which the veil is removed and our ostrich feathers ruffled. Time during convalescence is best spent looking at some of these painful issues. After all, our cover has been blown, we need help; we must find a way to ask for it.

e. Smoking

There is only one thing to say, and that is *don't*, and if you do then *stop at once*. Smoking has a definite and proven damaging effect on heart muscle. If you've never smoked, or only had the odd cigar once a month, then don't start smoking. If you have been smoking more than five cigarettes per day, by stopping after a heart attack you are cutting down your chances of having another attack by *seven times*. (See section on smoking in Chapter 7.)

So how do you give up is our next problem. My husband smoked sixty cigarettes a day before he had his heart attack; he used to light up before he got out of bed in the mornings. After his heart attack he was given large doses of MORPHINE, and he lay in this drugged state for a fortnight, apparently, he said, not wanting a cigarette at all, such was the quality of the MORPHINE. Later he was on VALIUM and this helped him through the withdrawal stage of giving up smoking. I'm not recommending this, as I don't know enough about it, except that this drugged state helped what must have been an addiction. It was hard to maintain no smoking and I know that he occasionally longs for a cigarette now, but the evidence is so overwhelming, and if you have gone through the agonies of giving up even for a month, it's crazy to subject yourself to it when you stop again. So find a way that helps you to stop: hypnotherapy, herbal cigarettes, deconditioning yourself of the addiction to nicotine. When the urge to smoke becomes unbearable go out for a walk, practise meditation, turn on some music, have a swim, dig the garden if you are up to it, have a glass of iced water or a very hot peppermint drink. If smoking has been your answer to getting rid of tension, try other ways to reduce your tension . . . some of the relaxation methods, positive thinking, reading, even sighing and yelling, but something that does not draw you back into the destructive spiral of smoking. Collect help from family and friends, don't have cigarettes in the house and avoid friends who are heavy smokers until you feel more safe.

f. *Angina*

WHAT IS ANGINA?

Angina means pain around the heart, and may or may not be associated with coronary artery disease. People describe their angina in different ways: "It's like a tight band around my chest." "It's like a great crab landed on my chest." "It's like a great hand clutching at me, stopping me breathe." And people's angina pains last for differing times from five seconds to up to four minutes; and come at varying times – climbing stairs, cooking lunch, lying in the bath, walking across a room, whilst hearing bad news, being emotionally upset or feeling anxious.

If you have had a heart attack you may never have had angina, but only experienced pain during your heart attack. Conversely many people suffer from angina without having had a heart attack. With the aid of the coronary arteriogram it can be seen that two patients can have the same degree of narrowings in the coronary arteries, but one patient may have severe angina and the other only fleeting pain or none at all.

WHAT TO DO IN IMMEDIATE TERMS

You can see from the above that angina is an individual phenomenon with its own individual pattern of occurrences. If you get angina the *first task is not to panic*. Panic and fear increase the effort of the heart – raising pulse and blood pressure – and stimulate neuroendocrine arousal. This accentuates the pain felt and prolongs it. At the same time we tend to breathe shallowly when we panic or are afraid, and may hyperventilate, putting even more pressure on the cardiovascular system. *Relaxation* – either lying down in a sloping L position with your back and neck supported by cushions, or sitting comfortably in a chair, together with concentrating on *regular, abdominal breathing* (see Chapters 1 and 7) will help the episode of angina to pass as quickly as possible. Some people are helped by using visualisation techniques. For example: close your eyes and imagine you are in a favourite or secret, private place. If nothing specific comes to mind, imagine a place, let whatever image comes to you come freely. Put yourself right in there and explore all around yourself through touch, sight, smell or sound. If you find yourself on a mossy bank, touch the softness of the moss; if you are at a Beethoven concert, hear and absorb the music; if you are in a honeysuckle garden, breathe in the fragrance of the flowers slowly with your regular abdominal breaths; if a beautiful flock of swans swim before you on a lake, rejoice in the sight of them. Give yourself fully to the experience and allow your heart to calm and sort itself out. You will be helping it by not being overtaken with fear and worry.

LONG-TERM MANAGEMENT

If angina attacks persist you will need to seek advice from your general practitioner. A practitioner with an holistic approach will look both at your physiology and at your personal make-up and lifestyle. Attending only to the physiological model – to the known risk factors associated with coronary artery disease – does not help angina. Cutting down on cholesterol, stopping smoking or losing weight alone has little effect. But a good plan for the management and self care in the control of angina can be extremely effective. In the chapter on medical treatments I explain the acronym SABRES used by Dr. Nixon's team at Charing Cross and invented by them. Attending seriously to each of the areas outlined by SABRES will help you in the long-term management of angina. *Monitoring* your episodes of pain will help you to ascertain whether or not there is a pattern to them. When monitoring, write down in a small notebook the time and place where angina occurs, anything else that is going on, who is around and, most important, what you were thinking prior to the pain coming on. After a week you will be able to see if there is any pattern to the attacks of pain and to take the necessary action. What happens to us, our attitude to this and where our thoughts take us, sets the climate for our feelings. Negative thinking can bring on negative feeling such as impotent anger which turns inwards against ourselves, a sense of hopelessness, despair and self doubt, as we 'think' badly about ourselves in a given situation. Negative thinking over a long period of time becomes a kind of internal nagging that undermines self-esteem and coping abilities. The combination of blood chemistry changes mentioned through-out this book in response to internally aroused feelings, and the sense of trap and defeat, can make angina more frequent than it need be.

When you know what situations or thoughts make you most

vulnerable to angina you have more control over it. Knowing that situations are likely to be difficult and will call on all our reserves helps us to plan ahead. If you are going into a difficult, taxing situation, whether it's exercise or confrontation with another person, know that this is likely to be the main call for energy from the heart, so do not fill your day with other, equally taxing events. Stop before angina comes on, and certainly when you feel that pain might be beginning. It is a mistake to carry on – hanging curtains or bicycling to work are examples I have come across – when your body clearly isn't ready. Stop until you are completely free of pain and properly rested before going on. Just as the diabetic patient has to prepare himself with the correct dose of insulin and also know what situations take most demand on his blood sugar levels, so a patient who has a tendency to angina can be prepared with learned skills. In severe cases where anginal pain hampers everyday activities, nitroglycerine is given to put under the tongue during pain to increase the blood flow to the heart muscle. With practice and patience it is possible to control angina successfully enough to lead an ordinary life.

g. High Blood Pressure (Hypertension)

Through its rhythmic pumping, the heart builds up pressure inside the arteries which moves blood along into the tissues. When the heart muscle contracts, it speeds up the flow of blood and this registers as a systolic pressure (the top figure in blood pressure readings). When the heart relaxes, the pressure on the flow of blood relaxes and this is registered as the diastolic pressure. Blood pressure rises naturally as our arousal mechanism is switched on after we wake in the mornings and begin our day, and it rises in response to different stimuli – fear, a sudden noise or shock, strenuous exercise and continual struggle at work or other activity – and it tends to rise with age. The normal range of blood pressure readings are within 140/90 when measured regularly over a period of about one month with accurate reliable equipment. Mild high blood pressure is considered to be between the range for 'normal' to 160/95 up to 105. This mildly high blood pressure does not put someone at risk from heart attack unless they are male, over forty-five and they smoke cigarettes. It is advisable, however, if you find your blood pressure to be consistently raised, to seek help with relaxation techniques which can help to bring the levels down. Blood pressure is diagnosed as being moderately high when the levels reach between 160–180 over 105 to 115. Above this level is considered to be severe high blood pressure, which, if prolonged, can produce changes in the tissues of the heart, brain and kidney and cause disease in these organs. *High blood pressure alone is not a disease* and doctors are of varying opinions as to the effective and appropriate treatment.

From the studies of the Medical Research Council working party* of mild to moderate hypertension, the recommended first approach to treatment of hypertension is to look at the individual's approach to life and his or her lifestyle, and see what personal contributory factors are pushing up the pressure. Redundancy, problems at home, periods of prolonged stress can put up blood pressure and this can respond to the 'human' approach, suggesting relaxation and attention to stress-producing factors in the person's life. James P. Henry† of Southern California School of Medicine describes two responses to external stimuli or life events. One is the dominant, aggressive fight-or-flight defence of status and territorial control response, requiring effort and arousing the sympathetic adrenal medullary stimulation; and the other is the subordinate response of dejection, loss of control, submissive, helpless response of internalisation and immobilisation stimulating the pituitary adrenal-cortical axis. Helplessness develops when a person perceives their situation is uncontrollable, for example when lifelong expectations fail to be met, close friends move or die, or a familiar support system breaks up. This can occur with bereavement, redundancy, during long illness or after accidents, where there is a sense of giving up of personal expression, a bottling up of feelings and a sense of dejection and despair. Both these responses to what happens outside in our lives produce chemical changes in the blood which influence a rise in the levels

* Medical Research Council Working Party on mild hypertension (1986).

† J. P. Henry. "Understanding the early pathophysiology of essential hypertension," Jan. 1976.

of blood pressure. Effective treatment in terms of personal training and guidance depends upon a correct diagnosis of the type of response to life events the person is engaged in. A person experiencing the more dominant fight or flight response triggering off more effort, output and arousal will need to be helped to understand the appropriate use of effort according to what is going on in his life and how to relax effectively. Someone who gets in a state because they feel down, dejected or hopeless will need to be approached with an emphasis upon raising self-esteem, self-assertion and enhancing past coping skills.

Once the personal aspects of someone's life are understood, they can learn relaxation techniques or meditation, and the importance of sleep and rest. After the concentration of human aspects involved in raised blood pressure, which require the skills of a GP, occupational therapist or nurses trained in the holistic approach to treating blood pressure, a diuretic drug such as Diazide may be used to bring the blood pressure down. Obviously there is no point giving medication if the reason for the raised blood pressure is not attended to. But medication may assist the process of personal control, whilst the training and learning process is taking place. Some doctors use beta blocking drugs as a desperate measure to bring down blood pressure if it is severely high, but the side effects of such drugs (drowsiness, heaviness, sickness) can be distressing, and drugs are of limited value if given in isolation without trying the personal, individual approach, and offer no preventative value in terms of heart attacks.

Some patients who have a heart attack never have high blood pressure. If high blood pressure was a contributory factor in your heart attack, then taking a close look at what is pushing the pressure up is going to be very important. Learning to take your own blood pressure and monitoring it can be a way to find out what times or events in your day are pushing up the rate. If your rate comes down after sleep and rest, then you can see that it is something to do with what is happening in your day and your attitude to this which is pushing it up. Some hospital staff, occupational therapists, nurses and GPs are specially interested in the human response involved in raised blood pressure and it is worth finding out who in your area can help you. There is sadly a shortage of nurses trained to help people in this way and this is possibly due to the way that public funds are spent in the health service. Funds tend to be for equipment and surgery rather than for training staff to help patients to learn to stay healthy through their own efforts. This is the conflict I mentioned at the beginning of this book between looking at the disease model of illness which must be cut out and cured, and the holistic model of health where people are encouraged to stay well and not wait until they are sick before seeking help.

If you have moderately high blood pressure:

1. Consult your GP and ask for his help.
2. Learn to take and monitor your own blood pressure.
3. Find out what it is inside you that contributes to pushing up the rate. Begin making priorities in your lifestyle – what is really important to you?
4. Value rest and sleep and place them as a priority every day.
5. Learn to relax properly and to meditate daily (see sections on relaxation and meditation).

h.   Meditation and Relaxation

MEDITATION

For the stress of everyday living, for anxiety, for tension, we should concentrate our energies on meditation rather than medication. Meditation, practised daily, offers us a powerful link between our minds and our bodies, which we can train ourselves to use beneficially and which can be a lifesaver.

In Eastern countries meditation is practised as a part of life. Before the decline of practised religion in this country, many people took part in regular, ritualised prayer and singing, chanting and self-examination, which acted as a kind of meditation. Unfortunately we have come a long way past this and most of us have only too little time for meditative processes. We tend to turn instead to instant remedies:

television, tranquillisers, cigarettes, alcohol and slot machine games.

It has been proved medically that if a form of meditation is practised regularly and thoroughly, this has a positively beneficial effect on the chemistry of the body. Blood pressure goes down, blood sugar levels go down, cholesterol levels decrease, adrenalin levels decrease. The more these techniques are practised, the more powerful is the body's stronghold of reserve. If an anxiety-making situation occurs, the person who has practised his techniques will know instantly to use them; they will have become automatic, and he will be sufficiently in touch with his body's reactions to know when the danger signs occur. We have all heard of the Indian Yogi who can walk on a bed of nails, reduce his heartbeats and breathing to virtually nil; we may dismiss it as Indian trickery, but it is an extreme example of the way in which we can use our minds to have an effect on our bodies. In a heart attack it is your body that is sending you messages – one big message. It is possible now for you to reverse this process, to start using your mind to give something to your own body, to be in charge, to assist, to beneficially work to getting your body physically healthy and then remain so. This is a much more powerful drug than anything manufactured in a chemist's laboratory.

You will probably be aware of the effect of tension and anxiety on your body . . . your pulse rate (and blood pressure) rise before an important occasion. Sometimes we can actually feel and think we hear our hearts pounding; when we are new and inexperienced, faced with a new situation or a public situation like making a speech or giving a demonstration, our blood pressure can rise from 120/90 to 180/130 and our pulse rise from normal (about 70–80) in most adults, to 150 or more. Less conscious are the areas of emotion, anger and turbulance inside, which raise our pulse and blood pressure without us knowing. People have been surprised that in talking about relationships which are causing them anguish, their blood pressure has risen significantly to warrant chemical change in the blood. If you can look at an average day in these terms, you will be able to judge just how much you are putting your cardiovascular system under pressure. At first, avoid tension and anxiety-making situations if you can. At the same time, armour yourself with the self-help techniques of meditation and relaxation, and spend a little time exploring which situations make you most tense. You now have a test barometer, your heart, for ascertaining which these are. Meditation practised for 20 minutes twice a day actually increases your energy level and efficiency, and your awareness; it acts as a benevolent stimulant.

Siddha Meditation Seminars, organised by Dr. Malcolm Carruthers, teach SIDDHA MEDITATION, a spontaneous form of meditation which has proved to be an effective treatment for anxiety, giving benefit to the body as well as the mind. Dr. Carruthers also organises a programme of AUTOGENIC TRAINING which, in eight training sessions, teaches people a form of self-hypnosis. This has been proved to have a strong effect on the body, bringing down blood pressure, lowering blood sugar levels and producing such inner calm as to have a spontaneous effect on the body chemistry. Books and addresses are at the end of this book.

There are also classes in TRANCENDENTAL MEDITATION in many places. Try looking in your local telephone book, or write to their head office and ask for your nearest teacher.

RELAXATION

Meditation and relaxation share one thing – they require you to claim time and space for yourself, to be alone with yourself. If, by the end of your rehabilitation period, you are able to practise meditation twenty minutes in the morning, and twenty minutes before 7.00pm, and half an hour of relaxation in the middle of the day, you are well armoured to deal with everyday stress.

There is a chicken and egg situation between relaxation and moods. Sometimes, if someone is very pent up with emotion, they are unable to relax under any circumstances. They need to express their feelings first. The reverse is also possible – if someone is by nature moody, relaxation can prevent their mood from becoming 'stuck'. When someone cannot sleep, and they have learnt self-hypnosis or relaxation techniques, they are better off putting this into practice than pacing up and down and swallowing pills or whisky and possibly making themselves more awake than before.

The wonder of relaxation techniques is that you can take them anywhere, secretly in the store of knowledge in your person, and you can whip them out in a crowded room, whilst waiting for a train, sitting in a bus, even while you are being nagged or shouted at by someone. It is a wonderful secret armour to both guard your right to a bit of time and space, and within which you can act to soothe your wrinkles and creases. The first thing is to give yourself permission to relax, and the time in which to do it. There is no point whatsoever in putting it off until you have done all the other things you have to do, or leaving it until last because you are so busy. The whole point of it is that it becomes an integral part of your day; it becomes something you do for yourself, as important as brushing your teeth night and morning. If necessary, you do need to be able to say to your family, or at work: "I just need ten or fifteen minutes to myself". Into that time you put what you have learned of relaxation. There are many techniques, and these are best learned from a professional relaxation expert. Your doctor might know of one in your area, or you could learn yoga breathing, meditation techniques or self-hypnosis. Relaxation requires you to take the phone off the hook and ask someone else to listen for callers. This is your time, all yours, and you don't have to share it with anyone.

It is very important to think about our space and boundaries, and to discover where they lie for us. Many of us don't have any at all; we let other people come crashing into our space most of the time and wonder why we feel crowded or harrassed. Watch any business executive who goes into his office. He is immediately surrounded by people who want his attention, his signature, his ear about something . . . they all press themselves forward to get his time before he has had a chance to see what his day looks like. Many women live with this kind of thing all the time. They can't go to the loo or answer the telephone before that eternal cry "Muuuum" comes large as life and their privacy is interrupted. As a society, we are very bad at it – it's quite amazing how often you see people quietly reading a book on a park bench or in a train and another person tries to engage them in conversation, as though their reading was an affront to the rights of others who are not reading, and an invitation to engage the other in conversation. We all need private space – we need to honour it in others and to claim it for ourselves.

There are many books on relaxation techniques which you can buy in most bookshops, but the very best way is to learn from an experienced teacher. It is never a waste of time to have this education and it is well worth keeping up what you have learnt, even if you feel perfectly relaxed and feel the discipline to be unnecessary. The main idea of learning relaxation techniques is that you remain relaxed all the time, thus not allowing your body to become overloaded and out of balance with strain. Betty Parsons, who has had many years of teaching relaxation to pregnant mothers and now to cardiac patients, describes the art of relaxation as using energy creatively, and uses the analogy of a bank balance to describe the body's energy . . . if you take too much out without putting any in, you get a rude letter from your bank manager, i.e. the body. Rather than waiting for the rude letter, it is wiser, more efficient, and, in the long term, life-saving, to use relaxation as part of your daily routine. A major shock such as the one just experienced should be enough to warn against the dangers of getting overloaded.

Here is one basic relaxation technique you can teach yourself: lie flat in a comfortable position, head supported, arms by your side, feet uncrossed. Take two or three deep breaths by allowing your diaphragm to be fully extended before filling your lungs with air, holding the breath when you have filled the lungs to capacity and then breathing slowly out again. Begin to relax your whole body from the toes upwards by imagining each part of your body, bit by bit, and as you hold an image of it in your mind, clench the part tightly together, hold it there, and then let it go, completely relaxed. Start with your toes, your feet, the balls of your feet, ankles, calves, knees, muscles of the thighs, buttocks, abdomen, chest, the muscles along your back, up the spinal column, that place in the small of your back which often feels painful, your shoulders, tops of arms, elbows, forearms, hands, clench and unclench them, the back of your neck, head, your forehead, jaw, cheekbones, eyes, let them sink further into their sockets, relax your ears, your mouth. Go through each part of the body as though you are discovering it for the first time. When you have gone through all of this, your whole body should be completely relaxed. Remember to clench your muscle and then relax it, to keep your breathing steady and to give over your complete concentration to what it is you are doing, and not to give half an ear to whether the telephone rings.

HATHA YOGA is practised widely throughout this country now and there are many good teachers. In many towns, the adult education centre offers courses and groups and some large firms organise yoga teaching for their employees. This seems to be a growing habit now that more and more people are realising the benefits of learned and practised yoga relaxation. You learn breathing techniques which are invaluable to you in the everyday sense, and you can get into your yoga breathing wherever you are and whenever you feel tense or anxious. The yoga exercises have a wonderful healing and calming effect on the body, ironing out all those kinks and creases that put us into awkward and inefficient postures and causing us pains in our muscles, aches in our joints, stiff necks, aching shoulders and stiff, immovable jaws. It sounds wonderful, doesn't it, and it really does work. Learn it, practise it regularly. Join a regular group if you can. This will help you to form and structure your learning time rather than leaving it to do when you have finished whatever you have to finish – which is often never. Don't put it off.

i.   Moods and Depression

Depression . . . most of us suffer from this at one time or another, and it is a word which we often pluck from our vocabulary and use to explain away our vague feelings of unhappiness. Some people are intolerant of depression, especially if they themselves have never felt depressed, and it gets dismissed with sentences like "pull yourself together"; "count your blessings" and "look on the bright side". There are many kinds and shades of depression, but feelings of depression are only too real . . . "the black dog", it is called sometimes. It cannot be rationalised away, or charted in logic, but has its own particular momentum, its own tide along with which one is carried, often much against one's will. When we are depressed, we are forced to look inward, to consider our inner selves. A heart attack is a body blow, and none of us can sustain a great blow and pass on as if nothing had happened. Depression is often the way in which we are forced by our psyches to examine what has happened to us.

For the sufferer of depression, there seems no way in which the flood of black, often frightening, feelings can be stopped from enveloping us like a shroud. People who try and jolly us along, however well meaning, appear hearty and insensitive, their behaviour overdone, exaggerated. We sink lower into the pit, unable to meet others in their jollity, hating them for what we see as their crude probings, and ourselves for not being able to mask our misery. We can only go with it, not fight it.

Some people feel that by 'giving in' and not fighting they are being weak, that they will never get over it or come out of it, but remain trapped. What people usually mean by 'fighting' is to ignore their symptoms; pretend they aren't there and 'snap out of it' like their friends tell them to, or they fight with pills, with too much activity, too much alcohol, too forced a smile. This is one way of coping, but it does not get at the source of the depression, rather it masks what is going on underneath.

There are times, of course, when we do benefit from the help of medication. This can be an important support when we are depressed but, ideally, it is best used together with more communicative ways of looking at what is happening to you – talking to someone, writing down your thoughts on paper, painting pictures of the images you are holding inside you.

There are times when we have to carry on in the everyday sense, masking our depressed feelings as best we can, and some of us are very good at doing this. It is amazing how clever people can be at hiding their feelings, especially if they lead a busy life, so that when they break down or become more severely ill their friends and associates are amazed, cannot understand it, never saw it coming.

So, if we recognise ourselves from the above, let's look at how we can do a mixture of what suits us best.

Depression after a heart attack is usual; the severity will depend on what was going on in your life before you were ill. Bouts of depression are healthy, our natural way of making us stop rushing about or masking our feelings, a way of getting us to consider our inner lives: who we are, what we want.

Sometimes kindness, acceptance, warmth, and the continuing loving routine of home life are enough to hold a period of depression until it passes. There is a fashion today to remove feelings of depression at all costs, by drugs or therapy. But there is a function that depression needs to offer, which should not be overlooked.

Underneath depression there is often repressed anger, and what more natural feeling in the world would there be than for you to feel angry with yourself, with the world, with everyone, because you have had to suffer a heart attack? If this rings a bell, see if you can offer such feelings a vehicle for them to be expressed. If you have someone close to you, tell them how you feel. What is it you feel inside? If you feel angry, do you also feel guilty for being angry? What would you like to do with all this anger? Throw something, break something, kick something, punch something? Whatever it is, act out these feelings when you feel ready, and strong enough.

Feelings of anger raise many anxieties and many fears because our society does not encourage the use or expression of anger as a natural place in a relationship and, indeed, in life. I'm sure one of the reasons why there is so much vandalism is that there are no reasonable channels for expressing anger. It all gets bottled up under the niceties we encourage our children to accept as sociable, and which our education calls civilised, and it has to come out in extremes by ripping up train seats or slashing telephone boxes. But if you are depressed and maybe angry for a reason, those feelings need to be expressed. Maybe you need to kick a football, plunge a fork into the soil, pound the sofa with your fists, wrestle with a towel in the bathroom; whatever; saying any kind of swear-word as you do so . . . everyone has their own expressions.

It may be that you will need to do these things alone, having got permission to do them. But you do need to focus your energies on what it is you are mad at, however vague this appears to be at first. More than likely it will be your body or the illness itself. Understanding, which is vital, will come later . . . you will never accept any of the deeper considerations of heart disease if you do not recognise your anger.

Bouts of expressing anger, particularly if it is unfamiliar, are often followed by tears, and these tears are of relief and compassion for the feelings that have been stirred up. There is a great deal of energy expended during these times and they need to be followed by something constructive. Put the feelings down somewhere, keep a journal of them on bits of paper, use anything that is at hand – it does not have to be 'constructive' – you don't have to show it to anyone. A walk, a sleep, watching a film, tidying a cupboard, can help the aftermath of strong feeling; it can form a 'holding period' during which, or after which, you may have a realisation or new thought. Some people write letters when they are angry, putting down all the vehemence they feel is choking them insiae. They don't post the letters, of course, but the writing has formed a channel for the emotion, or you may want to act something out, having an IMAGINARY CONVERSATION, using an empty chair as the object of what it is you need to tell another.

DRAWING and PAINTING are other ways; maybe you can work in THREE DIMENSIONAL TEXTURES: clay or plasticine, or carve away at sticks or pieces of stone. Being aware of, and writing down, our DREAMS may also help during this time. Keep a notebook and pencil by your bed so you can write your dreams down before they slip away. Dreams are the language of the unconscious, there to inform us, through images, of the state of our unconscious. Sometimes dreams do not need interpretation but stand alone, their power acknowledged and recognised, and over-interpretation can take away their magical quality. Just acknowledging their place in your life is the first important step, giving them space and letting *them* speak to you. When you have written down a dream, particularly if it had a 'charged' quality, see if it will speak to you about what it means. The important thing is, if you have an image of a house say, then ask yourself what a house means to you – is it where you live, are you trying to sell one or change one; what kind of house is it – yours, someone else's – whose? Do you like it, and so on; is it from the past, what are your associations with this house, how old were you; what was going on at that time in your life? What is the dream attempting to show you now – what are the similarities between what is being shown in the dream and what you are experiencing now?

Look at the time, colour, if any, size, place and nature of the dream and ponder on what it is showing you. Dreaming is a sign that our unconscious is actively trying to communicate with our conscious mind. Natural balancing forces operate within the psyche to help us to restore balance when we have become too one-sided or 'stuck'.

Dreams can be frightening, contain powerful material and we may fear them. They are too important to ignore and the consequences of ignoring their messages may be even more frightening. Remember that symbols offer many interpretations and are totally subjective. Dreams of death may not mean that you are to die, literally, but part of you is to die – the ego-ridden, over-conscious side, so that the birth of another part of you may take place – so we need to ask ourselves what death is for us, an ending of what? No one can tell you what your dreams mean. Your dreams may be amplified by someone experienced in working with dreams, but they are yours, they are precious, they have their own special magical quality. Let this live. Depression needs to be accepted as part of the important process of healing. Within depression, the psyche is having time to rebalance itself, the ego is being forced to stop taking such absolute control.

What we mean by the ego is that part of us which copes in the world, the part of us that gets on with living, that presents us to the outside world. Ego-consciousness tends to be rather 'one-way', self-centred, seeing one order of things, it puts itself first. We need an ego through which to function and express ourselves, but when the ego becomes too fixed, too inflexible, it takes over in a demanding and selfish way, not letting other things through, either from the inner or outer world. Big egos are rather narcissistic and, in their self-seeking blindness, they are unable to consider a flexibility of being. We tend to think of ego-consciousness as being that which takes us through the first half of life, when we are involved in the 'doing' values rather than the 'being' values. We go out into the world, establish skills, gain position and money, friends, family, property, things, and we fulfil the function of the ego. If this becomes crystallised, it becomes like a prison cell in which the self (our inner being) is trapped because this other part of us has different values. Our self links us with another order in life, with that which is beyond logic or rational understanding, but which 'knows' about life, about what we feel and what we want. We may not have been in touch with this side of ourselves since childhood. One of the ways in which we may rekindle some of this 'being' side of our natures is through play and unstructured activities, and details of this will be discussed in the next chapter.

Depression, as well as being the symptom for buried anger, is also the trigger point for discovering ways in which we may get a better equilibrium for ourselves, a greater sense of 'wholeness' where our ego, which is necessary to function in life, and our inner self, which is concerned with belief, love, creativity, wonder, a sense of being at one with the world, are intertwined successfully with each other and one does not grow at the expense of the other. It is in this way that we go into the second half of life with a greater sense of awareness about what life means to us, or what it can mean from now on, and a greater sense of a link between past and present. We are then in touch with collective forces, life eternal – there is no other 'security' than the kind we find in this way within ourselves.

Depression needs to be borne for a period, sometimes as long as two or three weeks at its worst stage, but if it seems to linger severely, getting on for months, then seeking professional help would be advisable. You may know of counsellors or therapists, or your G.P. may be able to suggest someone. There may be someone in the family or your circle of friends who acts as a kind of counsellor. Very often we are being counselled when we don't realise it. Friends who, by their natural warmth and understanding, accept us in whatever way we happen to be, have a counselling effect on us. Some people are able to talk to their parish priest, or the leader of a group they belong to.

There are several ways in which you can ascertain whether someone is depressed. He becomes listless, unable to concentrate for long, he may seem preoccupied, in a dream world. He may not want to do anything, complain of being tired a lot of the time, he may not sleep well, be unable to eat properly or digest the food that he does eat. He may have morbid thoughts, read morbid stories in the newspapers and his talk may be about dying or about people who have died or had their lives cut short by serious illness. The feeling you get is that a stranger is living in their body and this is a very distressing experience. These symptoms may range in their severity.

It is very hard to see someone you are close to become depressed, and it is also very threatening when you feel that you cannot reach them. If you can accept that depression is a natural occurrence after a major illness; that it is healthy and can be healing; that it will not last forever (even though it may seem like forever); that depression contains some very vital links for your patient to discover between the outer and inner limits of his being; that it can be, underneath all the pain, a valuable and enriching process for him, you will be greatly assisting his passage to recovery. Many of us rush ourselves or our children or family off to see a doctor the minute they appear depressed, and are greatly comforted by the offer of medication, and don't stop to wonder why the depression happens in the first place; whether it has any value, can be used creatively and usefully. Depression in someone we are close to is a great test of our love for them. If we can overcome our own fears and the nag of inconvenience or irritation that depression brings with it, we will be greatly assisting our partner back to health. But if you feel that the depression is becoming too severe, too heavy for your patient to hold himself, or if you become aware of serious suicidal feelings or morbid obsessions with death, do not hesitate to seek professional help.

j. *Thoughts of Death*

It is only reasonable that you will ponder on the fact of mortality. It is an extremely shattering thing to come face to face with this kind of reality for the first time. You can hardly fathom it at first, and are just aware of an acute sense of fear and confusion. It is as though life stops, and there is no clear way of going on. Everything you have known before gets shaken up, reproportioned, revalued. Many of the things that have contained great excitement or thrill pale in the light of this experience. Possessions become as worthless; achievements appear less important; some relationships become shallow or superficial. It is a great plummeting down to the realisation of one of the fundamental principles in life; that its ultimate goal is death. Elizabeth Kubler Ross writes: "Death is still a fearful, frightening happening, and the fear of death is a universal fear, even if we think we have mastered it on many levels."*

If you have had a heart attack, you cannot fail to concern yourself with the prospect of death and you may perhaps have come close to it during this experience. You will also wonder at the concept and what it means to you and you will value what you have all the more highly because of the experience.

You may react to your feelings about death in many different ways. You may become depressed, as we have talked about earlier; you may act indifferently, but be inwardly searching for some answers, puzzling over the next move, and you may 'test' your ability to stay in the world by overdoing activities, deliberately going against doctors' orders or close friends' wishes and entering a kind of race against death.

My own husband came out of hospital, where he had been for a month, and immediately got on his motorbike and careered up the road. I stood in the middle of the road in an

* *On Death and Dying*; Elizabeth Kubler Ross, Macmillan (1969)

attempt to stop him, but he swerved and went on. He ran up and down the stairs, he stayed up late and he had bouts of drinking far too much. This lasted for about three weeks and appeared to be something he had to do that was beyond any rational argument or persuasion. It was the most terrifying three weeks of my life. Having seen him through a heart attack and all those weeks of patient balancing of drugs and treatment, rest and stillness, it seemed ironic that he should immediately risk the possibility of being put out in a puff of smoke. I understand now what he was doing, but it is a very difficult thing to watch.

There must be, in every man suddenly suffering from a heart attack, when he appeared to be in good health in every other way, a sense of outrage, a sense of having the rug pulled unfairly from under him. This must stimulate a very male attempt to enter into what he might consider a fair game . . . pitting his wits against those of another in order that he may win or lose. In some ways a heart attack is a cheat, a blow below the belt because you didn't see it coming. To vie with traffic is like putting your fists up to fight a proper fight, face to face.

If you are watching all this, the philosophical way is to accept that there is nothing you can possibly do to alter the way that things have to be for your spouse or patient, if this is the whim he decides to follow. It is his contest between himself and himself and it can be argued that if he loses the race he needed to do so in the first place. Even if he were to read the above paragraph, he wouldn't see it as rationally as you or I might be doing now. It would not appeal to this kind of man's needs. He needs to have the experience, he needs to win this particular round, and then he might settle down to doing something about improving the quality of the life he has been given. There is no way that this kind of energy can be bottled up and processed nicely into something less threatening. So all you can do on the outside is to watch and bear it, accepting this frightening side of his needs and to think of it all as part of the recovery process. My own husband eventually got himself put back into intensive care after a bout of overdoing things (only this time it was overbreathing) and it was only after this that he let go of all his previous fantasies about survival and decided that he would put his energy into life instead of against it.

So, if you are pondering on death and what it means to you, have a look at how you were feeling before you had a heart attack. Can you recognise now any kind of struggle within yourself? Was there a part of you secretly wishing to die? Had a bit of you given up, gone on automatic, waiting for something to happen? Is a heart attack your way of being given permission to end something – in your life – something to do with work, a relationship or a private inner struggle you've never recognised? Do you secretly long for death, see it as a release from your problems, or are you in fact ready to die, feel that your earthly work is finished?

I have heard people say that death, for them, is very seductive. One or two people who are consciously ready to die, who have already embraced the meaning of truth, life and death in a full way have no fear of death and they work towards it, fully conscious. It is a natural extension of life, the goal in fact, of life.

There is a difference between being consciously ready to die and accepting the process when it occurs, and unconsciously struggling with life and death issues at the expense of your own body, perhaps again unconsciously, seeing death as the only way out. Think about where you are along the path of life and death. You may feel that death would be a cheat, unfair, too soon, you are not ready and your brush with death a sobering, frightening reminder of the price you pay for ignoring bodily messages or messages from life.

Is this, perhaps, a time for us all to contemplate our belief system: what we believe in, what we hold dear and true, what we value? Why are we here and what for? In thinking of this, are there things you need or wish to do that you have not begun to do or get started upon? Things to do with your particular mission in life, things that might consolidate your place on earth, your meaning for being here, and thus help to make death a more understood, reasoned and welcome goal of life at the appropriate time?

k. Play

Naked apples, woolly-coated peaches
Swelled on the garden wall. Unbounded
Odour of windless, spice-bearing trees
Surrounded my lying in sacred turf,
Made dense the guarded air – the forest of trees
Buoyed up therein like weeds in ocean
Lived without motion. I was the pearl,
Mother-of-pearl my bower. Milk-white the cirrhus
Streaked the blue egg shell of the distant sky,
Early and distant, over the spicy forest;
Wise was the fangless serpent, drowsy.
All this, indeed, I do not remember.
I remember the remembering, when first waking
I heard the golden gates behind me
Fall to, shut fast. On the flinty road,
Black frosty, blown on with an eastern wind,
I found my feet. Forth on a journey,
Gathering thin garment over aching bones,
I went. I wander still. But the world is round.

C. S. Lewis, (From a collection of his poems, edited by Walter Hooper, published by Harcourt Brace Jovanovitch).

Do we ever give ourselves time to return to the unbounded, wonderful oyster-like state in which we spent a large part of our childhood, where wonder, fantasy, stories and images held a special quality, a spellbinding capturing magic? With one or two exceptions – people whose childhoods were totally deprived of any kinds of freedom, with no experience of love or touching – most of us have some good childhood memories we can call upon. Perhaps we can remember something wonderful happening, like being given something we really wanted, finding a robin's nest, creeping out at night to watch for ghosts or Santa Claus. And those long uncharted days and nights when we had no 'oughts' or 'shoulds', or were totally involved in a particular game, knitting or a book, or watching tadpoles develop. Even long into adolescence there are similarities in terms of the use of time; those long nights of talk and exploration, sitting together with peer groups, airing one's views, sharing thoughts, spontaneous going with whatever happens in the moment. These are all examples of the process of playing, when we do not consciously strive to achieve anything specific, or try and have something to show for our time, to justify our use of it. We go with the unknown, with whatever happens. We allow ourselves to have unstructured time.

How do you play now? What kinds of things do you consider play? We tend to think of play in terms of organised games or activities and this is, indeed, one form of play, but things which become too highly competitive do not count as play – they might start off as play but become caught up as an extension of the ego and are subject to that control. Some competition is natural and healthy and exists within us always. It is when we become slaves to it that it is potentially harmful. Games might be your way to play . . . outdoor sports which you enjoy, not minding what happens: tennis, golf, squash, walking, hiking, riding. If you find that something which began as play has become too competitive, too hard work, see if you can get in touch once again with some of the feelings you had when you first began it; look again at whose choice it was originally. Indoor playing might be painting, sculpture, drawing, sewing, writing poetry or music, making music for yourself or to share spontaneously. Cooking, gardening, making things, can all be play if we have this attitude to them, if they remain fun for us and are something quite different from perhaps the work we have to do every day. Maybe we like to act, dress up, go to the theatre or cinema, socialise with friends or make a party.

Play should be something we hold very special and which we give to ourselves as a gift for a period of time, however small, most days. The way in which we play will, of course, be relative to the sort of lives we lead. Going to an exhibition with a friend would be play to someone who worked in an office all day and rushed out at lunchtime to buy dinner and home afterwards to cook it. Running along the sand in a pair of shorts would be play to a businessman who wore a suit all day and worked in an office. There is another kind of play which has no structure or shape around it in the form of games or activities. This is the kind of play we engage in when we let ourselves go.

Maybe in sex, in laughter, with good company, with wine and good food, when we allow ourselves to be carried away by an occasion, a grand event, a special day or happening . . . this is something we can enjoy alone or together. The royal wedding had an extremely powerful effect on people. We were able, for once, to be carried away with the idea of the fairytale prince and princess gliding off in perfection and happiness. Something archetypal was touched and we all felt it, we all were touched by it, even the most hardened cynics of the monarchy. What happened was nothing to do with being royal, or a nation gone commercial. We all carry within us an idealised sense of romantic or ideal love, an ideal state of being. When we get a glimpse of this, we get stirrings of something quite profound. It releases in us, even if for a second, some confirmation that we are not alone, that we share much on a collective level, if only we may know it and receive it. This 'knowing' is letting go of the order civilisation has made upon us, and sinking into being in touch with something original and timeless about life that no one can sellotape up into boxes or program into computers. We get in touch with this timelessness and joyful sense of collective sharing when we play.

If you do not know how to play – I had to learn it late in life – experiment with letting go, with not watching the clock, feeling you have to be useful, or account for the way in which you have spent time. Walking is quite a good way to start because you have space and time to be with your thoughts and dreams. Let yourself dream, daydream, for at least ten minutes twice a day at first. Don't try and stop yourself judging it a waste of time, but indulge in it and see what happens. In order to do this, you need to put your ego and superego elsewhere, together with all those voices that tell you that daydreaming is bad for you and will never get you anywhere. You also need the space for daydreaming. When you are in the bath, or out walking or preparing a meal, digging the garden, before you switch on the television or radio, telephone a friend or engage in talking to someone, have a few of those precious minutes for yourself, for your particular daydream.

You can see that playing is really a state of mind rather than anything else, and one which so often seems to be sadly missing from our everyday lives. Some people we can easily recognise as being naturally playful: they have a strong sense of the 'child' in them, and are often 'intuitive' types who are in touch with the 'knowing'. If you know someone of this type, watch them for a bit and see how they become playful, what it is about them that appears relaxed and has fun easily. How can you also brighten up your day in such a manner?

Playing has, I believe, a vitally important function in our everyday lives. Knowing how to play and giving oneself the unstructured time for play opens up for us those unbounded channels through which our natural creativity expresses itself. Not necessarily making or producing things, but the spontaneous creativity of being a human being in whatever way that may express itself for us. Being able to play makes us more communicative, more sensitive to others and our surroundings, more able to laugh and more creative in our everyday lives.

Frances Wickes writes: "The sand painter knows that not one grain of sand must fall except in accordance with the ancient pattern. He knows, too, that his work will be wiped out at the setting of the sun, but in the ritual act he re-energises (re-creates) spirit in himself and in his tribe. Transformation, which is the purpose of the creative spirit, moves in original concept, in re-animation of the image, or in recurrent ritualistic repetition. For the eternal images contain a spiritual energy that transcends the limits of time and awakens new life in the one that serves them. They move from wholeness and re-create wholeness."*

1.   Work

This is often the first question people ask . . . "when will I be able to get back to work?" Doctors' answers vary, and are often vague, because they will not know how convalescence proceeds until it does, and getting back to work depends on how you feel and how much you are able to do. A rough guideline, if all goes

* *The Inner World of Choice*; Frances G. Wickes, Coventure (1977).

well, is part-time work after six to eight weeks, working towards perhaps full-time work after three months. It is important to have some time schedule to work towards and many men respond to this well as they are used to working within a structured shape. But it is equally important to have a loose structure, to give you room to stretch and breathe.

Letting go of the kind of work structure we have been used to is very difficult for many people and they have an enormous struggle to cope with their time and the shape of their day. Boredom occurs when you are at odds with time. Some of the activities outlined in the previous chapter may help. Try and use this period also, for a re-appraisal of the nature of the work you do. How much do you like what you do? How much did you have to do with choosing it in the beginning? How did you get started? What would you do now had you the choice? How much has your work contributed to your illness?

On the positive side, people have told me that they are better managers after having a heart attack, more patient, more prepared to listen, more relaxed, more open to change. They have learnt what pushing against the system can do, and how destructive it can be. If they like their work and are committed to it, their after heart attack time can be more useful and productive than before. Again on the positive side, if you recover well from your heart attack, airing and ironing out some of your life's problems and making even small changes for a healthier way of life, you are likely to be back at work and working well within a very short time. Some people have told me that they keep the fact of having a heart attack very quiet at first, fearing that it might be seen as a weakness, but tell people with some pride later on, when they speak from a body of robust health. Some people fear they might lose their job, or that someone might take their place while they are away. This is clearly a matter of great concern, and it is important that you, or someone with your interests at heart, does keep in touch with your place of work and gives them good, positive messages as to how you are faring, without jeopardising your period of convalescence, when you consider the nature of what is ahead of you. There is no point in rushing back to work too early, only to work badly and fall ill again. Make your position clear, make your job as safe as possible whilst you consider your options and get better. (*See also note 2 on page 208.*)

What if you are a long-distance lorry driver – one of the most stressful kinds of work there is – but you love it and can't wait to get back to it? You just want to do the quickest repair job on yourself that you can and get yourself back on the road. This may be against your doctor's advice and at odds with the statistics and information about behaviour leading to a heart attack. It may be too soon, and you know this but ignore it. Nothing can stop you. However much we may plead with a man like you not to rush back on the road, to take a quieter driving job, to consider your health at least until you are stronger, you are likely to push forward, all cries unheeded.

There comes a point where we have to accept that everyone is ultimately responsible for their own lives and their own choices. It is their lives that they gamble with and it is their choice to take risks. We can only offer knowledge and counsel and, however subtle or determined our efforts, each individual has to take our offerings or not, and this is up to him. There is nothing we can do beyond this point for it is not our territory. We have to carry on loving people for themselves, however this manifests itself. I imagine those who much love racing drivers and daredevils like Evil Kneivel live with this development of philosophy all the time.

If you pause to consider the above paragraph . . . dare you face the fact that your job may be killing you slowly? I write this with some concern because this is a tough thing to face, but maybe you have to. Facing up to this fact does not mean you have to rush into something else. Just acknowledging what your job is doing to you is enough at first. To stay with this thought and make a choice whether to leave it or not, is your second task, and to seek help with change, should this be what you decide, is the next task, and this may take some time. You may have to return to the stressful job for a short time until change is possible and maybe within your new-found realisations you are able to negotiate for better hours, better pay, more considerate time schedules. If you have decided to make a change, this decision alone will give you more energy, more relief, more space to experience yourself.

Another thing that a heart attack does do is give you permission to stop for a bit, and then to think about change, and there are many of us who need this kind of permission. "I sold my business"; "I went on to part-time"; "I took up golf/ painting"; "I moved into a smaller house/nearer the sea/my son or daughter". How often do we hear this said followed by the words "after my heart attack"? In terms of work, many men, and, sadly, increasingly more women, view having a heart attack as an achievement medal for hard work. "Look how hard I tried"; "how hard I worked" is silently stated. And after such a statement to the world, some people feel satisfied that they have fulfilled the requirements of society, or "them", whoever "they" are. They have proved themselves and can now relax and, at last, do what they really want to do. A man I know who had recently suffered a heart attack said to me "Real men have heart attacks; quiche eaters get haemorrhoids". He had proved to the world he could run with the hare, hunt with the hounds in business, and now he could become a poet and eat quiche, haemorrhoids regardless. Some people do not feel satisfied with one heart attack but go on striving more and more against greater and greater odds with disastrous consequences.

If you are the female partner reading this, you may realise that the re-evaluation of a man's work is an important time for a woman also to look at what she is doing with her time. Have you thought about where you come in the order of things? How much of what your husband does has been stimulated by you, egged on by you? How much does your partner work in order to fulfil your ideals, your hopes, your needs, and how much do you do to fulfil these for yourself? These are hard questions and important ones, and it is important that you answer them honestly. You may have, unwittingly, been putting your own ambition onto your partner and be asking him to work this out for you, to carry it for you, instead of having a go at it yourself.

You may say that you have never had the opportunity to do anything about your ambition, and how could you, with a house to run and children to bring up, etc. . . . but think again now. How does what I have just said apply to now? A little soul-searching never does any harm and no-one is accusing you of doing wrong.

It is not wrong to have ambition, but it is cowardly to ask another to carry it out for you, because in doing this it is they who carry also the disappointments and the risks; it is they who suffer from failure or who have to deal with success. While the ambition may have been yours, the result of this has been his and you have been living vicariously. Think through. Did you push him on for promotion or object to it? Did you refuse to move when he was offered an opportunity to change the nature of his work? How much of his career have you been involved in; who do you know where he works; how much do you know of the nature of his day, what he has to deal with, the kind of pressures he is under? How supportive are you when he needs to talk about work?

How much of the style in which you live, the things that you do, holidays, clothes, children's education, hobbies, parties, gifts, have been instigated by you and fostered, and how much is your partner's? Some women say: "We'd never do anything or go anywhere, if it wasn't for me"; or "they've got me to thank for that", suggesting that it was a lone voyage that was sailed, and it probably was and might be a very good thing . . . but what of your partner's "not doing anything" . . . is it really idleness, or a genuine desire just not to do anything? . . . How much of this energy has been put into events which possibly have little significance when the energy might have been used in backing your spouse financially or in supporting what he is doing.

This isn't a time for blame or guilt; it is a time for honesty and for doing something to help the situation. Have a look at how much energy you have, and how you can use it together with your spouse to achieve some of the ambitions that you both have. You may discover that you want to live in the country, or in the town, or work together at a new project. You may find out that you would like to be the breadwinner for a while, if you aren't already, and your spouse wants to be a student. You might have too many animals, too many unnecessary expenses.

Granny might have been allowed to be too interfering; you may have too crowded accommodation or have not had a holiday for the last ten years. It may be the car or the journey to work; you may hate your old furniture, need a bigger window in your sitting room, have nosy neighbours that you've never been able to deal with. These are all practical considerations and you may have taken them for granted for years, never really facing them or talking about them, just becoming more and more weighed down by their presence. Now you have the time and the opportunity to explore your likes and dislikes together and to work out a compromise . . . maybe not immediately, but you can make promises to yourself in the future.

I met a man in hospital who was recovering from his third heart attack. He was a precision worker making spectacles, which was what his father had worked at before him. He came from Poland and settled here in the 1940's. His work involved the most detailed accuracy and he was always having to work to deadlines. He worked, hunched up in artificial light all day long. His greatest hobby was fishing, but his wife grumbled at him for being out on Sundays when she wanted him to mow the lawn and put up cupboards, and so he didn't go very often. He was a dapper and neat little man who sat neatly in his hospital bed with his long fingers tucked together in front of him. He didn't say much, but he wore disappointment on his face in the way that some people wear smiles. When I talked to him and asked him questions, he answered them by saying: "My wife . . . she likes", or "My wife, she's the one for tidiness", and so on. His wife seemed omnipresent. He wanted to give up his work so that he didn't have to use his eyes to such a fine point of order, but his wife's needs got in the way and he was too much programmed into her ways to resist. It seemed that, in his case, his wife had answered for him.

Work, for us all, should ideally not be a laboured drag through which we force ourselves to pass time. Sadly, for many, it becomes an evil necessity in exchange for money on which to live. I have idealistic hopes that the next generation will seek to change this and that, ultimately, work and leisure will become intertwined, part of life in a more wholesome, communal sense, with much less emphasis on financial gain and individual achievement and more on the quality of life for everyone as a whole. Maybe heart attacks in their increasing numbers are one of the symbols that will make a sufficient number of us hold up our hands and say "stop . . . this kind of living actually endangers life".

m. Loneliness

Has having a heart attack accentuated your feeling of loneliness? Feeling lonely is not the same as being alone. We can feel lonely in an unhappy marriage, in a crowded room where we feel we don't belong, on a beach where we feel fat, or with a group of long-standing colleagues who do not know that our spouse has just left us or that secretly we hate our jobs.

Are you afraid that now you have had a heart attack you have been branded as weak, that no-one will trust you in quite the same way again, that people will be afraid you might become ill on them or drop dead? Are you someone who cares very much about what people might think and whether or not they like you?

Have a look next at people you do feel that you are close to and at how much they matter to you, examine what they are like, how they behave, how you behave when you are together. Could you get closer, or is there something stopping you? Are you afraid of closeness: does it make you feel stifled, claustrophobic? Have you prided yourself on being a 'loner', only to find that there were times when you wished you weren't? Has there been something stopping you getting close to another person? Now that you have time to consider your life, would you like to change this, to perhaps have more real friends, become more intimate with someone, to feel a close link and to care and be cared for?

Perhaps when you leave hospital you have no-one with whom to share your convalescence. This may not matter to you, you may prefer to be alone with yourself and your thoughts. If it does matter to you, you might like to find someone with whom to share these feelings. You may never have had to ask for help from anyone before, and be shy of doing so. It may never have occurred to you that you might ever need such help and you therefore resent having such a need and feel angry at it.

There are, for everyone, times in life when human contact of a totally personal and exclusive kind is so very important. The first step is to ask. Ask the hospital social worker, counsellor, doctor who appears sympathetic, or a hospital visitor – most hospitals have voluntary visitors who come in especially to see patients who have no family or other visitors and they are usually people who are easy to talk to. One of these may well be able to arrange for you to be taken home or on to convalescence with them or someone else they nominate, and for you to have someone to talk to and be with during this time.

This may be your first experience of talking with someone about yourself. Through this experience you may feel like going on to make other contacts outside, to improve your communication skills for when you get back to work, or within your local area. It might 'break the ice' for you and help you to get started on a more social basis so that your life becomes more fruitful in terms of people, and less lonely and isolated. There are all kinds of voluntary organisations today which are well staffed and funded and in your area there may be one to serve your needs. You may well need only an introduction to the idea of wanting more company and to meet one or two people for this to make all the difference in the world.

If you do have family and friends, you will need them now very much. They can do a great deal to support you now, to encourage you, be cheerful company, and loving, nurturing companions. Illness is a time when you find out who your true friends really are. If you have such friends, let them be friends; there is no need to be lonely. You can help yourself not to be by accepting friendship and letting it in, allowing it to warm you, give you something. Perhaps this is the first time you have realised the value of friends and from now on are more likely to value this and to be a good friend yourself.

Ultimately, of course, we face life alone, making small, everyday decisions which we alone can make, and in facing our illness we do so alone in the privacy of our personality. This need not be a lonely experience, but merely an alone one. In learning to be alone, we learn to be more familiar with ourselves, our personalities and our more undefined 'inner' selves and responses. Hopefully through being alone we learn to like, love and respect ourselves more.

n.   Why? and what does it mean?

There is an appropriate moment, some time after the initial crisis which we have been so absorbingly involved in, when we may have periods of contemplation and introspection, when the question "What does it mean?" may arise. Most of us go about our daily lives never stopping to wonder on the meaning of life's events. But something as major as a heart attack, which shuffles so many issues around like cards in a pack, does merit some pondering and philosophical thought. If you are the type to look inward, you will want to sort out some answers. Some useful questions to ask at this time are:

"What has this illness and crisis forced me to look at?"

"What is the main question that has emerged? . . . Is it my relationship, work, money, a third person, the state in which I had been living, my standards of living . . . or is it something within the embrace of the personality, something to do with the body, or the mind, the emotions, with sexuality, with a deeply buried past, with a fear of the future?"

"Have I been opting out of something, avoiding something?"

There is an idea that has some support, which says we are all implicated personally in what happens to us. Obviously some accidents really are accidents and do just happen. But a heart attack, when it happens, has been brewing there inside the body for some time. It doesn't just happen overnight. Often the attack is the result of fifteen or twenty years of some internal difficulty which only becomes conscious after the body has been laid low and all these conflicts reach the light of day.

97

Many people do not realise how tense they are until they get a headache or one of their vertebrae goes "out" in their spine. Many people do not realise they are unhappy until they find tears pouring unexpectedly down their cheeks or see their reflection in a shop window. All of us harbour feelings of anger, fear, resentment, hurt and confusion that we are unable to express at the time they are provoked. Sometimes we can do little about the pressures we come up against and we learn to endure them because we can see no other alternative, but we do this at a cost. This cost is usually within our bodies. What happens to tension, emotional pain, frustration, anger, fear, when it cannot be expressed? Think of the adrenalin that pours into the stomach when you are afraid or excited . . . if it isn't used up in the "fight or flight" it was designed for, where does it go? What happens to the tension in the muscles and tissues when it is never properly released?

In our daily lives, many of us take risks; we spend a lot of time in danger or in nerve-wracking work, meeting deadlines, cutting costs, racing with competition, overloading ourselves because of budgets or because we think we are the only one who can take the responsibility or because other people give us this charge and we accept it. We may heave a sigh of relief when a particularly difficult feat is accomplished and think "thank God that's all over", but is it really all over in terms of what our bodies are carrying?

Have a think about what you have been asking your body to carry for the last ten or more years. Make a list of all the jobs you ask your body to do for you (including carrying around extra weight) and another list of what you give your body as a reward . . . proper food, sleep, relaxation, play and fun time. See if you can look at the resulting paper as you might a balance sheet, noticing if you might be overdrawn, how much you are in the red, and why you have got such a rude letter from the manager of this balance sheet. This will also help to give you some idea of what you need to do to repair the damage that has been done, and some idea of what you need to do to balance things up so that you don't get any more rude letters. Here is a list of stress factors which you might like to consider:

EVENT	SCALE OF IMPACT	EVENT	SCALE OF IMPACT
Death of spouse	100	Son or daughter leaving home	29
Divorce	73	Trouble with in-laws	29
Marital separation	65	Major personal achievement	28
Jail term	63	Change in spouse's work	26
Death of close family member	63	Starting or leaving school	26
Personal injury or illness	53	Change in living conditions	25
Marriage	50	Revision of personal habits	24
Loss of job	47	Trouble with boss	23
Marital reconciliation	45	Change in work hours	20
Retirement	45	Change in residence	20
Health problems in family	44	Change in schools	20
Pregnancy	40	Change in recreation	19
Sexual difficulties	39	Change in church activities	19
Gain of new family member	39	Change in social activities	18
Business re-adjustment	39	Small mortgage taken out	17
Change in finances	38	Change in sleeping habits	16
Death of close friend	37	Change in family reunions	15
Change in line of work	36	Change in eating habits	15
Argument with spouse	35	Vacation	13
Large mortgage taken out	31	Christmas	12
Foreclosure of mortgage	30	Minor violations of the law	11
Change in work status	29		

If you score more than 150 points during the last six months you are under stress and your chances of becoming ill are much greater than normal. (See also section d of Chapter 7 on the subject of stress.)

There is another kind of tension that exists within the human being which is concerned with the psychic whole of the individual. We come with two parts to us: our psyche and our soma. The soma represents the physical body that we are in, and the psyche that part which we do not see but which we sense embraces our mysterious whole, our soul or spirit, our underworld.

C.G. Jung believed that the psyche has within it powerful regulating forces in charge of the balance of our whole being. When we become out of balance or live in an extreme or lopsided manner, the psyche has a way of pulling at the areas

which have been neglected or repressed so that they come to the
light of consciousness in an attempt to restore the balance of the
whole. The psyche therefore sends messages . . . sometimes
through the language of the unconscious which represents itself
in dreams and images, or through the triggering off of events.
In this way we attract to us the behaviour or events that mirror
our internal needs so that we may have the opportunity for
balance. Often these opportunities go unheeded or the messages
from the unconscious unheard, and they return later on in a
more powerful, or even violent, form. Learning to develop the
kind of sensitivity to listen to the internal messages of our
bodies and our psyches is a life-long task, but one which leads
to the greatest sense of completeness and purposefulness in life.
In this way we go with life rather than pit ourselves against it.

If, perhaps, you have been avoiding something, or not facing
up to something and your heart has broken under the strain,
what can you do now about it? We have talked so far about
heart attacks granting one permission for change, being a cry
for help, a status symbol for the hardworking, and if any of
these points are uncovered and result in realisation and change
then so much the better. But what if there is something more
destructive going on; if you harbour angry feelings about
someone or something and want to punish them for making
you feel the way you do, but cannot quite find a way of saying
what you feel or doing anything about it and it gets turned
against yourself? Harbouring a lifetime's hostility inside your
body is destructive and dangerous and a heart attack may be
your warning. It may be the point at which you say: "It's me or
them" and make your choice. This is a problem that will not
keep, and when you are feeling stronger, more able to take
stock and make a few moves, try and make some resolution for
yourself on this question, hard and painful though it may be.
You could be helped by a skilled counsellor or therapist; you
may benefit from a more long term period of analysis to probe
more deeply what it is you hold within you that has gone sour.
You will certainly need support of some kind to help you to
come to terms with this factor in your life.

What you do want to avoid is getting into a situation where

you feel your only defence is in illness behaviour, so that the minute trouble comes along your body speaks up rather than your mind or your feelings. This is destructive for you and for your family and relationships. You can stop this process from developing by recognising it now, at the beginning, before it is too late, and take the responsibility for change.

Chapter 3

Digesting Medical
Information

a. *Digesting Medical Language*

A HEART ATTACK will plunge you into the world of medical
words, terms and jargon. While the doctors may explain to you
what they mean and show you diagrams and drawings, it is just
as well to go over these matters for yourself in your own time,
so that you can satisfy yourself as to what they mean. There
may be choices you have to make, perhaps together with your
partner, about treatment, especially surgery.

The first thing to grasp is the working of the heart itself. The
heart is a hollow, cone-shaped, muscular pump, made up of the
thickest strongest muscle in the body. It is about as big as the
clenched fist of the person who owns it and it is situated to the
left of the breast-bone with its widest part uppermost and its
bottom, or apex, forming the point of the cone shape around
the fifth and sixth ribs. The heart is divided into four muscular
chambers, each of which is separated from the others by valves.
Blood comes into the right side, is pumped through the lungs to
discharge its load of carbon dioxide and take in fresh oxygen
and is pumped out from the left side. VEINS bring blood *to* the
heart *from* the body and arteries take blood *away* from the heart.
The LEFT VENTRICLE, situated at the bottom left of the heart, is
the largest and most muscular chamber of the heart and is
responsible for pumping the blood around the whole of the
body as well as serving the blood supply of the heart itself. In
most heart attacks it is this area that is affected, in one of the
three coronary arteries that supply fresh blood to the heart
itself. Thus the word 'coronary'.

DIAGRAM OF THE HEART

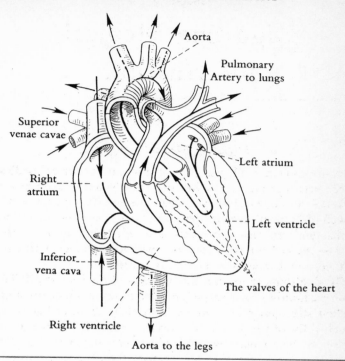

The LEFT and RIGHT CORONARY ARTERIES leave the AORTA and the left divides into two parts, the ANTERIOR DESCENDING ARTERY and the CIRCUMFLEX ARTERY. The anterior descending artery goes down bewteen the two ventricles and, together with the circumflex artery, supplies blood to the front and left side of the heart. The right coronary artery goes to the back of the heart.

MYOCARDIAL INFARCTION: Branches of the coronary arteries supply blood to the muscle wall. When a coronary artery narrows because of disease or plaque (a patch of deposit situated within the artery wall), a blood clot (THROMBUS) may form at the narrowest point where blood collects and cannot move freely. If this blood clot enlarges together with the increase in narrowing of the artery, it will eventually block the artery altogether, thus cutting off the main blood supply to part of the heart muscle, causing the muscle to die. This is called a myocardial infarction. When heart muscle dies it throws the work of the heart into disorder and puts a great strain on the rest of the muscle which has to take over the work of the part which has died. Often the heart enlarges to accommodate this. Eventually the damaged area forms a permanent scar which shows up on the ELECTROCARDIOGRAM or E.C.G. This is the machine with which you will now be familiar; it graphs the electrical activity of the heart as it is seen from different positions. The electrical activity of the heart concerns the heart beat and is monitored by the heart's natural PACEMAKER. This extremely sensitive series of NERVE BUNDLES is situated in the wall of the RIGHT ATRIUM. In emotional situations such as extreme anxiety, fear or excitement, the brain will stimulate these nerves, causing the heart to increase its rate to pump blood more quickly to the muscles of the body to get ready for 'fight or flight'. The blood supply for this system comes directly from the coronary artery branches, so you can see both how much work the coronary arteries have to do and how closely linked they are with the heart's electrical system. When the electrical system is damaged because of a heart attack the heart may go into what is known as FIBRILLATION (the regular beat is replaced by the two sides of the heart being out of synchronisation and pulsating irregularly) and a machine called a DEFIBRILLATOR will have to be used to restore the regular beat. A defibrillator is also used to restore the heart's electrical activity if the heart has stopped beating. Sometimes it is necessary to insert an ARTIFICIAL PACEMAKER to ensure the regular beat of the heart and this is quite a simple operation. Many people have artificial pacemakers for years and live with them very comfortably.

ARRHYTHMIA   is an irregular heart rate or rhythm.

HYPERTENSION   is simply high blood pressure and this condition may be free from symptoms. Persistent hypertension can cause kidney failure and heart attack.

You hear the word ATHEROSCLEROSIS a great deal and it should not be confused with ARTERIOSCLEROSIS. Atherosclerosis is a disease of unknown origin in which the inner layer of the artery wall becomes thick and irregular from the piling up of fatty deposits called ATHEROMATA. The disease develops slowly over a period of years.

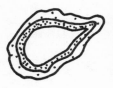 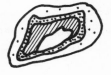 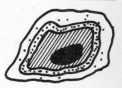

(i) Cross section of normal artery

(ii) Arterial opening narrowed by fatty deposits

(iii) Arterial opening blocked by blood clot

Formation of atheroschlerotic deposit in artery wall*

Sometimes the scar tissue left in the heart muscle after a heart attack weakens under the pressure of the constantly beating heart. This causes an ANEURISM, or bulging of the wall, and it can be removed by surgery. An aneurism can form in one of the chambers of the heart itself or in one of the main arteries within the heart, particularly the aorta, and many happen without any infarction taking place.

ANGINA PECTORIS is the name given to the pain felt around the heart, similar to the pain of a heart attack, which is brought on usually by exercise, and is relieved by rest. It is a symptom of oxygen deficiency and *not* a sign of impending doom. The severity of anginal pain bears almost no relation to the extent of the disease in the coronary arteries. There is now a well-recognised group of patients who have anginal pain but with completely clear coronary arteries.

CORONARY INSUFFICIENCY occurs when there is not enough

* *The American Heart Association Handbook*, Dutton (1980).

blood supply to the coronary arteries and the left ventricle.

OEDEMA: presence of abnormally large amounts of fluid in body tissues.

EMBOLUS: clot which travels through bloodstream to lodge in a small vessel and obstruct circulation.

HOMEOSTASIS: state of equilibrium in which the chemical substances and other components of the body are in balance.

HYPERLIPIDEMIA: abnormally high concentration of fats in the blood.

LIPIDS: fatty substances, including cholesterol, triglyceride and phospholipid, present in blood and tissues.

MITRAL VALVE separates left atrium from left ventricle in heart.

PERICARDITIS: inflammation of the lining (pericardium) of the heart.

P/S RATIO: ratio of polyunsaturated to saturated fats in the diet.

PULMONARY OEDEMA: condition associated with heart failure in which left ventricle does not pump adequately, causing fluid to accumulate in the lungs.

SYSTOLIC: phase of heart's cycle during which heart muscle contracts to pump blood to the body.

ADRENALIN or epinephrine, is a hormone secreted by the adrenal gland which has a profound effect on blood vessels, heart and bronchioles in the lungs. These actions are classified as alpha and beta. Beta effects stimulate the rate and contraction force of the heart. Alpha reactions contract arterioles and raise blood pressure in large doses of adrenalin.

ALVEOLI: small air sacs in the lungs from which blood receives oxygen and gives off carbon dioxide.

ANAEROBIC REACTION takes place in the absence of oxygen.

ANASTOMOSIS: connection between two vessels or grafts.

ANOXIA: condition where there is absence of oxygen.

ARTERIAL THROMBOSIS: blood clot formed within arterial system.

ARTERIOLES: small muscular vessels formed from branches of arteries.

ATHEROMA: deposit of lipid or fatty material and cholesterol within artery wall which may narrow or block the lumen of an artery. The most common cause of heart attacks and strokes.

CYANOSIS: clinical condition caused by too little oxygen in blood, characterised by bluish appearance.

DIASTOLE: the phase of the heart's cycle during which it relaxes and the chambers fill with blood.

HYPERVENTILATION occurs through 'overbreathing'. This results in there not being enough carbon dioxide in the blood. Tingling sensations are felt in the feet and hands with sometimes loss of feeling altogether. Dizziness is also experienced. One quick remedy is to breathe into a paper bag to recover the lost carbon dioxide. Hyperventilation can cause coronary spasm.

AROUSAL: internal stress registering as being 'on edge', alert, preoccupied, vigilant, which can become so all-consuming and out of proportion that we cannot take in reasoned argument or helpful suggestion. A state produced by our internal coping mechanisms to presumed external stressors.

ANGIOPLASTY: a catheter is passed into the coronary arteries in order to compress soft narrowings and make a wider space for blood to pass.

ANABOLIC refers to a healthy unaroused state in which healthy functioning can take place.

CATABOLIC is the opposite to anabolic. Healthy functioning is impaired because of a high state of arousal raising blood chemistry changes – catecholemines, trigycerides, lipids, cholesterol – blood pressure and pulse rates. Often produced by prolonged and intense fear, anxiety or anger.

b. Tests and Cardiac Equipment

After a heart attack your doctor or the hospital you have attended will want to carry out tests to ascertain the extent of coronary damage and to find out whether surgery is necessary. These tests and what they entail are usually explained to you before you have them but they can be a frightening experience if you have not been fully informed what to expect. It is useful to know that most medical technicians who run these tests are not qualified to tell you anything about what happens during the tests or the results of the tests. Their reticence and silence can be very annoying and frustrating if you are not prepared for it. Someone I interviewed described his frustration as he saw himself on the television screen in front of him, did not understand what it all meant and none of the technicians in the room would respond to his queries. When, under pressure, the technician did mutter something about all three coronary arteries being either blocked or narrowed, this man came away feeling very depressed. In fact, most of us have narrowing of the arteries as we get older and in his case his consultant cardiologist reassured him that his situation was not serious, did not need surgery at that particular time, and he could have saved himself a lot of anxiety if he hadn't pressured the technician for an answer. A technician is responsible for getting clear information, and the cardiologist for interpreting it, and it is important to pay attention to the rôle of each one. It is never good to listen to information or advice from people who are not qualified to give it or from whom it is inappropriate to pass on opinions. You and your family will save yourselves a great deal of worry by listening to the one person you have decided to trust.

An ANGIOGRAM is an x-ray of the heart and is performed by the injection of a radio–opaque dye into the blood system so that the outline of the heart's chambers may be seen and photographed. The dye is injected by means of CARDIAC CATHETERISATION, when a CATHETER (small tube) is inserted into the FEMORAL (leg) artery or the BRACHIAL (arm) artery and gently pushed along towards the heart so that the dye may be released. In cases where there is a suspicion of damage to the heart valves, the catheter is threaded through the heart itself. There are many variations of the kinds of tests done in this way according to the initial diagnosis of the condition. All the tests are done by extremely well-qualified technicians who are also doctors, in sterile conditions, and a local anaesthetic is given before the insertion of the catheter. Understandably, these particular "invasive" tests can cause great anxiety but they are well proven to be safe, are always done under supervision in a hospital, the patient rests afterwards for about twenty-four hours, and they are the most accurate way of seeing what damage the heart has sustained after a heart attack.

Other tests include a STRESS TEST in which an E.C.G. is taken during and after specific levels of exercise to determine the heart's exercise tolerance level. It can also disclose a disease condition which may not be evident at rest, but becomes apparent under stress.

ECHOCARDIOGRAPHY is a new technique in which ultrasound waves are beamed into the heart, reflected back onto a recording device and then processed into an image. This allows a doctor to view the movement of the heart valves and chamber walls and to examine the condition of the tissue.

HEART MONITORING. When a patient is in hospital after a heart attack, he will probably be connected to a heart monitor where the electrical activity of the heart and its pulse rate are shown on the oscilloscope (like a television screen). You will see that he has four soft pads on his chest linked by wires to the screen. Sometimes, in cases of palpitations or other chest discomfort thought to be associated with the heart, a patient is put onto twenty-four hour monitoring by tape. This involves his carrying a small tape recorder on a belt around his waist which is attached by electrodes to the chest. Each time he experiences some discomfort he writes down the time and details in his notebook which is then put together with the graph of the electrocardiagram after the twenty-four hours. This is a useful piece of research equipment to find out what happens to the heart during a normal twenty-four hours.

c. *Surgery*

The question of surgery can only be answered after detailed discussion with your doctor and the specialist cardiologist, who will have reviewed the results of your tests and medical history together with the present state of your health. The most common and successful operation is CORONARY ARTERY BYPASS GRAFTING.

CORONARY ARTERY BYPASS GRAFT

When the condition of one or more of the coronary arteries is rigidly blocked and this is not treatable by angioplasty, an operation can be performed to bypass the blocked area using veins taken from the leg or thigh, or the mammary artery from the chest. The surgeon will work from the angiogram film to decide where he will attach each end of the bypass and how many vessels should be bypassed – up to four vessels can be bypassed in this way. The operation has a very high success rate in this country and in America where it has become very common indeed. A word of caution needs to be expressed though. Sometimes arteries can be narrowed due to the effect of prolonged stress and exhaustion, sleep deprivation and hyperventilation. These narrowings are called dynamic narrowings and can respond to sleep and rest. If, however, the arteries have rigid narrowings which do not respond to sleep and rest or a change in lifestyle and the narrowings are a threat to life, then surgery will be recommended.

Most surgeons take time to explain what they are going to do and go through the operation in as much detail as the patient and his family require. Again, it is important to ask, to find out what is going to be done, if you want to be totally clear about it all and to avoid unnecessary fear and anxiety. Some people, however, do not want to know these details but prefer to leave it all to the surgeon and not to have to think about it. This quite surprised me in several of the men I met who wouldn't have dreamt of buying a house without a survey or putting money into a venture without doing their groundwork! In matters of the body some people are very passive or so frightened they deny interest. But someone in the family should know what is happening. It is useful to be rested and relaxed before the operation, to give the body as much restorative power as possible, particularly if you have been leading a busy, stressful life up until the operation date. You are less likely to have complications after the surgery if you are well rested beforehand.

PREPARATION.   A nurse will explain the procedures of the intensive care unit and make sure that one close relative is told what to expect. The whole chest and each leg are shaved completely (you feel as slippery as a seal) and you have an antiseptic bath. There is no food after midnight if the operation is the following morning.

PANIC.   It is not unusual to feel the stirrings of anxiety or panic just before being taken to the operating theatre. It would be surprising if you were not to feel strongly about what was about to happen to your body. Men particularly, who tend not to think much about their bodies, can get a flood of feelings when the great weight of realisation hits them ... will it hurt? ... will I be able to cope? ... will I survive...... will anything go wrong? If you are supporting a patient through this experience, reassurance and encouragement will be of great value, as will your quiet constant presence. It is very comforting to know that someone is gunning for you, that someone cares enough to want to stay close by.

AFTER THE OPERATION.   The first two days after a heart operation are spent in intensive care under the supervision of a team of specially trained nurses. This is nursing teamwork at its very best. Usually one nurse is assigned to a particular patient for the duration of her shift. After the operation, which takes about four hours, the patient is on a ventilator machine which breathes for him for about seven hours until the heart has adjusted to its new vessels and is ready to take on the work of working together with the lungs. Patients have a blood transfusion in one arm and another drip feed of glucose and saline in the other arm. Several drainage tubes coming from the wound in the chest cavity will connect to bottles placed under the bed. A catheter relieves urine from the bladder into a plastic bag which is strapped on the side of the bed. Patients are very drowsy after this long operation and are given pain-killing drugs, such as Omnipon, to relieve the pain from the sternum, which has been opened in order to operate upon the heart. There is also some pain from the legs where vein grafts have been taken. Sometimes patient's feet are wrapped in foil to help create warmth because during an operation the entire body temperature is reduced to between $24°$ and $32°C$ – a cooler body needs less oxygen. After about two hours – but this varies from person to person – the patient will begin to come round and usually feel the discomfort of having a breathing tube in his windpipe. He will gradually feel the atmosphere of the intensive care unit, which is a very busy place on operation day. Machines bleeping from time to time, computer screens flashing, ventilators wheezing, and the nurses' voices as they check observations every ten to fifteen minutes. Some people find intensive care very noisy. There is, of course, permanent daylight and if there is no clock on the wall, it can feel a timeless, endless, rather disorientating place to be in. Fortunately, much is being done now to remove these confusions and to make people feel as comfortable as possible, and visitors (close relatives) are able to come for short periods. Many people say that they remember very little about what happened in these two day. Two women I talked to had halucinatory experiences, one seeing the nurse as a grotesque spider.

After the intensive care period, patients are cared for in the cardiac wards. By the time they leave the intensive care unit, all their drip feeds and drainage tubes are removed, and they may only be attached to a monitor for the first twenty-four hours in the cardiac department. It is truly amazing to see your husband, wife or close friend sitting up in bed eating ice cream just three days after major heart surgery. If all goes well, going home day, from the surgeon's point of view, is sometimes after eight days, but much depends on the circumstances at home and the general attitude and well-being of the patient.

Aftercare after major heart surgery is very important. Not only has there been a tremendous shock to the body and psyche, but for some people the fact of surviving and just being alive is a major amazement. Everyone, after an operation like this, needs guidelines for convalescence, and in particular some kind of containment for the euphoria that often follows the bypass operation. It's easy to understand why some people feel that having come through a heart operation, got new vessels, they can get cracking immediately, doing exactly what they want, rushing to catch up with all the things left behind in the period leading up to the operation when healthy functioning was absent. If impatience and time urgency were dominant features before the operation, they will obviously play a role in convalescence.

Be patient at first. You need to allow enough time after an operation for your body to heal properly and for you to get used to knowing what your body needs at different times. Goal-orientated tasks for convalescence can be inappropriate and defeating. There is no 'set' time when the body 'should' be ready for certain activity. What is important is that you learn to recognise what you *can* do, and what you may *not have* the stamina for at any particular time. If you have a warm bath at 10.00 am, answer a difficult phone call at 10.30 am and drink a hot cup of tea at 10.45 am, your body may be at its limit of effort-making for the next 15 minutes, and anything else needs to wait until the body is rested and restored enough to take on more. This is known as *pacing the body*. If you rush too quickly to get through what you feel should be achieved in a day, you will get overtaxed and will collapse, cross and defeated. Concentrating on breathing, pacing, and saying 'no' when appropriate, even under hospital routine pressures, will establish a strong pattern for a healthy convalescence. It is hard to realise that even getting dressed is tiring at this time. Just travelling in the car from hospital to home, just seeing family faces again … it all requires effort and all this puts a demand on the heart.

PAIN.   The sternum scar will hurt for several weeks, particularly when you cough or turn on your side. This gets less and should wear off within four to six weeks.

MOOD CHANGES.   Something not often written about is the variety of mood swings after a heart operation, said to be the result of being on a heart-lung machine. People who've had the bypass operation report feeling depressed and edgy afterwards, but not often feelings of mania incoherence, but the families of patients do recall the latter. Their beloved one may seem disorientated or even a bit deranged, may talk rapidly or repeatedly about something quite unconnected, appear somewhat frenzied and manic. People report their spouses being excessively angry, hostile, nasty for a time after the operation. For most patients, these episodes pass and must not be taken literally or personally. It is possible that whatever was a personal 'tendency' before the operation, is exacerbated by the process of surgery and the post-operative shock. It may be worthwhile looking at the mood in terms of content for this may be something which needs attention. For example, if there was anger before, which was repressed, this may come out as pure rage; if there was obsessionality, this may appear as a kind of paranoia. Both may be an extreme sign of what has been lurking around for a while and may need looking at.

CONVALESCING. The first two weeks, after the return home to convalesce, are spent resting and walking, but with no lifting, driving or strenuous activity. Again, pulse taking is useful because it indicates what the heart has reserve for. The convalescent period is just the same as that recommended after a heart attack, with the added dimension of the painful healing sternum. You may have to sleep on your back for a while or need more pillows. And, of course, the big difference overall is that the heart has new vessels, and people report feeling better in general health immediately – circulation is better, breathing is better and there is usually freedom from angina pain if this was marked previously. Sometimes some anginal pain remains and this is discussed separately on pages 65–8.

The operation is so successful that people become bypass bores! There is no evidence that the operation prolongs life, but it certainly improves the quality of life.

Any reading that you can do on this subject, and a list of books is included at the end of this book, will be helpful if it develops your understanding. It would be foolish to read too many different opinions which are conflicting and cause confusion. At best you can begin to understand the physical work of the heart so that you know what medical people are talking about.

The other most helpful knowledge to have is an appreciation of the way in which the work of the heart is directly linked to stimuli coming from the brain which, in turn, are triggered off by behaviour which is governed by the personality. A diagram might look something like this:

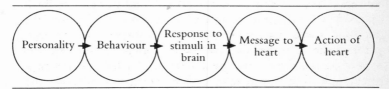

Personality → Behaviour → Response to stimuli in brain → Message to heart → Action of heart

When you have been able to put medical and physiological facts together with what you are already aware of about your personality you will have a pretty good grasp of which situations to avoid and which to encourage in future. This is one positive step in the direction of dispelling the myth that heart attacks are the act of some unknown murderer, who steals life before its time is truly up. This myth is perpetuated by fear and ignorance and it spreads merely those two things and causes unnecessary anxiety and suffering.

d. Medical Treatment

Medical treatment begins the moment you are diagnosed as suffering from a heart attack. You will be on complete bed rest with nursing care and, most probably, carefully regimented drugs, according to the needs of your condition. There is an extremely large number of different drugs in use and their names and dosage vary from country to country. One or two might be worth mentioning here.

BETA BLOCKERS such as BETACARDONE and INDERIL act upon the

beta adrenoceptors of the heart in order to slow down or "block" the level of stimulation which releases substances such as adrenalin and increases the tone of the sympathetic nervous system (the system dealing with the "fight or flight" mechanism we have talked about before). This blocking of the receivers lowers the heart rate, helps to keep blood pressure down and control rhythm disturbances. Beta blockers are used during intensive care treatment and may also be prescribed after you leave hospital. There are many experiments going on at the moment to determine the full value of beta blockers but so far they have marked a great advance in the treatment of coronary artery disease. It is important, however, not to rely solely on the workings of beta blockers to reduce the level of stress to the heart. Far more fundamental is the level of change within the habits and behaviour of the individual so that he is able to gauge his own tolerance levels, rest himself frequently and properly and lead a much healthier and happier life. (For more details on this, see the Human Function Curve in Chapter 7.)

DIGITALIS   This drug comes from the foxglove and has been used for over a hundred years. Its main use is in improving the efficiency of the heart contraction, thus enabling the heart to empty more efficiently. It has a direct effect on the electrical system of the heart so that its rate is slower and more efficient.

DIURETICS   assist in the excretion of fluids from the kidneys and help to take some of the burden off the circulatory system.

ANTI-COAGULANTS   reduce the ability of the blood to clot and may be prescribed to prevent blood clots developing in the legs or lungs after heart failure or arrhythmia. They do not "thin" the blood, but prolong the time needed for blood to clot and prevent blood clotting problems.

VASODILATORS   are used to relax blood vessels so that resistance to blood flow is decreased. The heart works no harder than before, but more blood reaches the tissues.

GLYCEROL TRI-NITRATE is a pain-relieving drug usually prescribed for angina sufferers to take before exercise that is likely to bring on pain.

Every medical practitioner will have a different method of medical care for his coronary patients. Some patients are cared for at home with a visiting nurse and doctor and in some parts of the country a "Hospital at Home" system has been encouraged. It has been noted in medical research that many coronary patients suffer great anxiety whilst in the impersonal confines of the coronary care unit or intensive care unit. The array of complicated equipment, rigid routine, endless rounds of medical personnel taking blood, recording pulses and pressures, taking notes and performing tests can actually raise a patient's arousal level at the very time he needs it to be lowered. If a heart patient is not in immediate danger and does not need scientific monitoring, it would seem that the best place for him to be is at home in his own bed, providing his wife and/or family can, and are willing, to cope with this situation. Naturally the family needs to have the support of their doctor and the local hospital, but there are reports that this system works well and patients recover fast.

One or two pioneering cardiologists, notably Dr. Peter Nixon at Charing Cross Hospital, London, are developing a medical regime for heart attack patients and for patients whom they consider are in an extreme state of exhaustion and arousal which, if not halted, will lead to coronary disorders. A period of complete rest and sleep, where the patient is prescribed VALIUM or a tranquillising drug, begins this treatment with patients simply sleeping for perhaps five or six days. Then the patient is encouraged to develop his self-help skills to help him become aware of his stress tolerance levels and to deal with them without recourse to drugs. He is taught to evaluate what in his life has caused a state of exhaustion and to discover ways of cutting down the stress-inducing components. He may be taught relaxation techniques, meditation, yoga, self-hypnosis, assertion techniques. He may be offered individual counselling if this is appropriate. During this time the emphasis is on good nursing care, rest, and on giving the body a period of complete relaxation so that its worn systems can begin to recover some of their strength.

There are still many fears and unknowns associated with the different treatments of heart attack and many of the new treatments are controversial. You may be assigned a cardiologist who believes in the knife at all costs, or another who is firmly devoted to a particular drug therapy, or another who uses sleep and relaxation. If your experience, in an emergency such as a heart attack, lands you in your local hospital casualty department, you have to go along with what is happening in the reality with which you find yourself. Later on, when you have time to question medical treatment and you feel that you would like either a second opinion or a change of treatment, you can embark on a different journey. It is just as unwise to question treatment which, at the time, has no alternative because it is all there is, as it is to accept treatment that both of you know in your guts is wrong for you, or which you find unmanageable. If, in the light of knowledge and experience, you decide to reject the ideas of your doctor, you need to have enough confidence and stamina to make your way toward the treatment you prefer. It is no good jumping from one idea to another, hoping to have the best of both worlds. In the beginning you have to be philosophical about where you find yourself and put positive energy into the situation, remembering, at the same time, that you do have a right to know what is happening to you, you do have a say in the matter and you need to be clear about airing your worries and fears.

SABRES*

S = Sleep – looking at the quality and quantity of the sleep that you have – how much your sleep is disturbed, unsatisfactory, full of worry and thoughts, and you wake still tired.
A = Arousal – that feeling of being constantly on edge, vigilant,

---

* SABRES is the acronym developed and used at Charing Cross Hospital in Dr. P. Nixon's unit. The staff in Dr. Nixon's team are skilled in helping patients to assess their need to pay attention to SABRES and are helped in areas where they are most in need.

alert and preoccupied to the extent of this becoming your every minute concern or obsession. Talking problems over with someone or seeking skilled help if problems are very great can help relieve this situation.

B = Breathing.

RE = Rest and Effort – try and develop a healthy balance of rest and effort according to the needs of your life and your heart.

S = Self-esteem – this means looking at how those negative inner voices undermine your everyday and trying to develop a stronger, positive input to counteract this negativity.

Chapter 4

Holistic Medicine and Healing Therapies

Through the centuries, healing has been practised by folk-healers who are guided by traditional wisdom that sees illness as a disorder of the whole person, involving not only the patient's body, but his mind, his self-image, his dependence on the physical and social environment, as well as his relation to the cosmos. . . . I would suspect that the whole imposing edifice of modern medicine, for all its breathtaking success, is like the celebrated Tower of Pisa, slightly off-balance.

Prince Charles in his speech to the British Medical Association in December, 1982.

IN RECENT years, some of the healing arts which had fallen into disfavour, with the rapid growth of science and technology, have been finding renewed respectability, as evidenced by the speech quoted above. 1983 saw the inaugural meeting of the newly-established British Holistic Medical Association, brought about because of growing dissatisfaction with the poor success rate of many of the technological answers to disease.

Heart disease is no exception. Many people are disturbed at the growing number of coronary bypass operations and pacemaker fittings which appear to have been performed when alternative treatments, less drastic, had not been tried. In the U.S.A., the bypass operation has become almost as common as appendectomy and a huge industry has grown up around this procedure, notably the growth of intensive care and coronary care units.

HOLISTIC MEDICINE is the opposite of this mechanistic approach. It looks at the person as a whole, not as a patient with a presenting illness by which to define himself. The holistic approach encourages a shared relationship between physician and individual as equals. It encourages the individual to take responsibility for his own health and it shares much of the Eastern view that health is something to be maintained rather than sought after after illness has set in. This is why it has a great deal to offer the person suffering coronary disease, because the contributory factors do seem to be rooted in the lifestyle of the sufferer. Rather like a counsellor or therapist, the holistic practitioner holds up a mirror so that the individual may see what has happened in its full context: for example external life and environment, family and past expectations, patterns of living, aspects of his mind, body, emotions and spirit, his belief and survival systems. The physician then interprets from his professional knowledge of the working of the body as a whole and suggests a method or approach to the disordered constitution. The approaches tend to be safe, do no harm and do not constitute some of the risks encountered by many of the more conventional methods.

The best use of holistic medicine is in an 'ongoing' sense. If you have not had a specific illness, but are concerned about your general health and suffer from minor irritations like colds, headaches, stress and tension, aches and pains, holistic approaches have much to offer you. After a heart attack, holistic medicine can help a great deal with maintaining good health, establishing a better balance of energy and creating a sense of well-being from taking responsibility for your own health. At a time of coronary crisis, however, it would be appropriate to consult a traditionally trained practitioner or go directly to the emergency department of a hospital. Here are some of the approaches you might find from a holistic practitioner.

HOMOEOPATHIC MEDICINE is well established as a healing art. It works on the principle that like cures like: a substance which in large doses produces certain symptoms in healthy people, is used by homoeopaths in minute, 'potentised' quantities, to treat people who are exhibiting exactly the same symptoms. The whole picture of the person's overall physical and psychological constitution, including past illnesses and treatments and family history is considered. A remedy is prescribed whose effect on healthy people, or in large quantities, is most similar to the symptomatic picture presented by the person in question.

The advantages of this approach include the avoidance of the use of drugs in large or toxic quantities, with the risk of unexpected and sometimes very dangerous side-effects. There is also no possibility of damage to the patient's immunological system by, in effect, poisons to the system.

Homoeopathic remedies are given to suit the individual and are not directed towards curing a particular illness. They are usually derived from natural sources such as plants, snakes and minerals. At one end of the spectrum they are useful as an aid to surgical treatment, involving the healing of wounds, or in cases of shock; at the other, they can also be used to unravel constitutional disorders of many years' standing, something which conventional allopathic practitioners rarely attempt.

If irreversible damage to the body has occurred, homoeopathic remedies can be palliative, but they are most valuable if used early on to prevent such damage from taking place.

ACUPUNCTURE is often used as an adjunct to conventional treatments and is particularly successful at treating recurrent pain. This traditional Chinese medicine works on the principle that disease is caused by an imbalance of Yin and Yang energies which can therefore be treated by correcting this imbalance. As the natural forces of the body return to a normal balance, the disease is then cured. The art is to be able to locate the specific imbalance in the meridiens, or channels of energy flow. Needles, heat, or pressure are then used to stimulate points on these meridiens. The acupuncture points represent points through which the maximum amount of energy may flow in channels to the particular organ represented by the channel. Disease is present when the flow of vital energy is blocked. Acupuncture can have a definite effect on the circulatory system and on the functional ability and efficiency of heart muscle. In his book *Acupuncture*, George T. Lewith writes that "80% of patients with angina have improved after acupuncture. A course of treatments is given, followed by booster treatments every four to six months". Acupuncture is less effective at treatment arrhythmias and raised blood pressure, but seeing an acupuncturist once a month to keep the energy flow of the body in balance might be a powerful antidote to becoming ill again, and is best used in this way, as part of the general care of the body and its systems.

HERBAL MEDICINES are often given in addition to acupuncture as many acupuncturists are also herbalists. Herbal medicine is on the increase in this country, and uses many different organically grown herbs as remedies. Once again the substance and the amount is given according to the individual's needs. There are herbal medicines for most complaints including raised blood pressure and angina. It is important to consult a qualified herbal doctor or herbalist, as herbs, although what one might call 'natural', are often also extremely potent and need to be used with knowledge and wisdom.

BACH FLOWER REMEDIES are best used when recommended by an experienced practitioner. They are all derived from flowers such as wild rose, star of Bethelehem, or larch. Some practitioners link each of the remedies to particular emotional and psychological difficulties, and are directed towards work on these. For example, some remedies have been found to work successfully on self-esteem, feelings of sadness and loss.

Some Healing Therapies

MASSAGE. This is a long-established custom and much the most personal of the healing therapies. Massage has many physical benefits, most especially its relaxing effect on the muscles and body as a whole and the release of energy flow and restoration of balance. There are different kinds of massage, from intuitive massage and the basic Swedish massage to the more dynamic forms of massage such as biodynamic massage and rolfing. The latter two are used in conjunction with specific emotional or psychological difficulties or body 'blocks'. When an area is reached through the deep massage and worked upon, often many significant memories are released and this process needs to be carefully monitored and held by an experienced person. Biodynamic massage has proved to be very effective in the treatment of such disturbances. For most general purposes, the more gentle form of massage is recommended. The very process of the 'laying on of hands' contributes to a feeling of well-being and intimacy with one's body, and the time given to lying still to be administered to is of great value to people who give only a little time to themselves in this very personal way. Massage can be learned reasonably easily and is a useful skill to have when a friend or close person is unwell or tense.

Often AROMATHERAPY and COLOUR THERAPY are used in conjunction with massage. AROMATHERAPY was a high art developed in ancient Egypt. Every flower has an oil, and each oil has a specific effect on different areas and organs of the body. Essential oils of many different kinds – flower essences, and pine, sandalwood, beech, frankincense, are chosen to suit the individual and are massaged into the part of the body in need of healing. Likewise, COLOUR may be used to surround the person, according to the nature and needs of the person. Both colour and smell affect the body as a whole, stimulating the visual and nasal passages and whole areas. Active imagination might well be used to concentrate upon an important area, and this may be combined with MUSIC chosen to have a healing quality.

ART THERAPY is a way of getting in touch with our inner images and symbols through painting and drawing. Often the individual is asked to produce an image or shape or colour for something, say his heart, and put it down on paper. There may be other images, or conflicting emotions which are troubling the person, which can be located in image form and 'anchored' by means of drawing. Often pictures themselves tell an intimate, internal story which often comes as a great surprise to the drawer. People often say "I can't draw for toffee" and are unclear as to the value of this kind of work, but it has been proved to be of immense value and is an extremely valuable tool which I use often in my own work.

ACTIVE IMAGINATION is the way we get in touch with our inner world and what it is trying to say to us. This leads to a rich unfolding of dreams and realisations, another 'order' within us and often is the key to our finding a lifeline of the inner kind, either a symbol or an idea. In their book *Getting Well Again*, Carl and Stephanie Simonton talk about getting in touch with our Inner Guide. There are also other figures such as our Inner Healer and Wise Person, which we may find through the process of imaging and active imagination and which may help us through the difficult journey of illness. Again, having an experienced teacher, therapist or guide is important because the images we find can be very powerful and a shape needs to be given to the process, a time limit and a guide or talisman to accompany us on such a journey.

REFLEXOLOGY or ZONE THERAPY looks at the body as an electromagnetic field. If that field becomes blocked in any area, imbalance begins and disease sets in. There are five zones in which organs, glands and nervous system are placed. The nerves which serve all these areas terminate in the ears, tongue, hands and feet. When pressure is applied to these terminal points, the specific area which the point serves is stimulated and this stimulation, by increasing the blood supply, releases toxins which are causing blockage and pain or dysfunction. Massage or pressure is given with the tip of a finger or thumb to begin with, followed by using more force or pressure, as this can be tolerated, sometimes with a hard plastic tool. Some of the conditions which respond to zone therapy are: arthritis, asthma, cystitis, diabetes, digestive problems, heart, blood pressure, hay fever, headaches, insomnia, prostate trouble, sciatica, sinus, bladder trouble and constipation.

Chapter 5

For Partner, Friend or Family: What if it Happens Again?

BY NOW YOUR knowledge of cardiac 'events' will have been extended and you will be familiar with medical or surgical procedures. One or two helpful people might have given you some hints on how to care for a cardiac patient once he's discharged from hospital and you have probably picked up quite an understanding just from visiting hospital and seeing what happens there. But the question "what if it happens again" will nag at you after your spouse or friend has returned and it is something that never goes far away from conscious thought. You cannot be at his side, waiting ready, in case of another heart attack. But you can know that if he does have another and you are there, that you will be able to act quickly and sensibly. Many heart patients fear every ache and pain that they feel and it takes time to adjust to being home after a heart attack and to get used to the fact that not every discomfort is going to be a major catastrophe. It is good for you, too, to get used to this and not rush into a panic the minute they have a pain in the chest or a fast pulse. Often you need to go through one or two 'scares' before you relax into a position of more confidence and can accept that a heart patient too has colds and gets toothache. However it is important that once we feel that someone is having a heart attack that we act promptly. The quicker our reactions are then the quicker a correct diagnosis is obtained and the quicker correct treatment is begun. Speed is absolutely vital and it really does make the different between life and death. When a heart attack is not acute – i.e. it does not happen suddenly and dramatically, resulting in immediate loss of consciousness, we do have time to talk with our 'patient' and help him to clarify what he is feeling.

It may be that you were not presnt when the heart attack occurred and are not sure what happens during an attack of this kind. There are many different ways in which a heart attack may manifest itself and often the symptoms of a heart attack are confused with other illness or disorders such as indigestion, stomach upset, tiredness. If, however, your partner has already had one attack it is unlikely that you will confuse these kinds of symptoms for you will be only too aware of his heart. Here are two examples of a first time heart attack as they have been described to me by different people:

EXAMPLE 1

He wakes in the night with an uncomfortable feeling some-where in his chest. He presumes it's indigestion, something he's eaten. (His mother always told him he bolted his food and you know that he's always in a hurry and doesn't eat properly.) You can't think of anything he's eaten that's unusual, unless it was something he ate in the office or picked up on his way home. He looks rather pale and greyish and you blame the bad light in the bedroom. You get him something – an alkaseltzer or indigestion tablet, but he feels the need to go to the bathroom himself. He may begin to belch a lot, he may vomit or have diarrhoea or all three, and this seems to confirm that it was something he ate that is causing the trouble. Gastro-enteritis, you think, like you all had on holiday last year. He may spend an unusually long time in the bathroom and he may be puzzled as to why his pain won't go away but seems to intensify. He comes back to bed and feels that it will go away if he can get back to sleep. You notice that he seems to be sweating, but he feels cold to the touch, and his hands and feet are very cold. He is wide awake, and disturbed about what is wrong with him. He keeps hoping that the pain will disappear, but it's not quite like anything he recognises or has been told about. You go through all the possibilities . . . gall stones, gastric 'flu, chill, ulcers, gastro-enteritis, hiatus hernia, heartburn, cracked ribs, pulled muscles . . . it feels like a combination of all these things. He looks grey, cold, clammy and ill. He cannot get comfortable and keeps turning about to try and find a better position. He is still belching a lot and may begin to get pains in his arms and up into his neck. As the pain seems to intensify it brings with it the disturbance of other functions such as breathing and flexing of the fingers. At this point you decide that whatever it is, he needs professional help. Only twenty minutes may have gone by since he first woke up.

EXAMPLE 2

He comes home from work feeling very tired. His face looks pinched and his complexion a little grey. His eyes look strained and seem to have sunk further into his sockets, leaving dark circles and patches under the lids. He seems to be forcing his breathing, as though he isn't getting enough air, and he takes deep breaths spasmodically. He is listless, rather depressed, has no energy, but seems unable to relax. He doesn't know where to put himself, but is in no particular pain. He will probably be unable to communicate exactly what is wrong with him and what he is feeling, except for a vague unease which he may dismiss as being due to the time of year, his overdraft, traffic jams or some other annoyance which has piled on top of him. He may have a certain amount of indigestion, or need to urinate often. He may have cramp-like pains in his arms and legs and a vague, heavy kind of pain in his chest. He may feel absolutely drained of energy. He may be in this situation for several days before he displays the typical symptoms of cardiac malfunction. Many people apparently do suffer mild heart attacks without realising it. But, if his behaviour is out of character and if you realise there are circumstances surrounding him which would tie in with the known risk factors involved in heart attack (see Chapter 7), or if what he says and communicates to you convinces you that all is not well inside his body, professional advice should be sought so that extensive damage to the heart can be avoided. The most vulnerable time for a heart patient is immediately after the attack, however small, when the heart is trying to restore some balance at the same time as serving the rest of the body. If diagnosis is not achieved or nursing care facilitated, complications within the function of the heart's own system can arise, and this can easily be avoided by an earlier decision to get medical aid. Details of what happens, or can happen to the heart, are dealt with in Chapter 3.

Different people respond differently to similar circumstances and each of us has our own particular way of describing an experience and choice of words for this. Having a heart attack has been described as:

"An elephant sitting on my chest."

"The ceiling has fallen down on top of me."

"I'm being twisted in half."

"Someone has put a hot electric cord around me."

"It's like being trapped in a vice."

"I'm on the rack."

"I'm being wrung out by a hand wringer."

"A horse has just left his shoe imbedded in my heart."

A second or indeed third heart attack should be treated in exactly the same way as if it was the first, unless you have special instructions from your doctor or the hospital. Here are some guidelines:

WHAT TO DO

If you have good reason to believe that your partner is having a heart attack, or even if you simply suspect it, you need to take action, and you can choose from the following as appropriate:

1   Telephone your G.P. If you are able to talk to him, or to another medically qualified person, tell them the symptoms as you have seen them, clearly and slowly. They will want to know what time the attack started, what kind of pain is being experienced, whether the breathing or pulse is rapid, and what is the colour of the skin. You may not be very good at taking pulses, and the pulse rate does not necessarily change during a heart attack, but it is useful to learn pulse-taking, as it is a reassuring thing to be able to do, both for you and your partner, in a stressful situation. If you know that your doctor will not be there, that you will only

get a recorded message, or that you will not be able to speak to anyone who can really help you, it is better to leave this possibility alone as it only wastes valuable time. If you do speak to your doctor he will either come out himself or recommend some other action to you, but whatever he does do will depend on how clearly you tell him what is happening.

2   Dial 999, ask for an ambulance and say that your partner is having a heart attack. Again, be sure to be clear about your address, your name, whether you live up a flight of stairs, or any other appropriate information.

3   If for any reason these two things fail or you know they will not bring about the result you want, try and get help from a neighbour or friend with a car, or get help to assist your partner into your own car and drive him to the nearest casualty department. Make sure that the hospital you are driving to does have a casualty department.

One thing is quite definite and that is that in the case of a heart attack there must be a medical diagnosis in order to bring about the correct treatment, whether this takes place in hospital or at home. You will need to decide which is the best, most efficient and quickest way of getting your partner to medical treatment.

WHAT YOU CAN DO WHILST WAITING FOR THE DOCTOR OR AMBULANCE

You have called for professional help and now your partner is your patient until help arrives. What can you do?

The first thing is to try and be as calm and relaxed as you possibly can, even if you don't feel it inside. Fear and panic are so easily communicated, and your patient will need all the energy he can get to help him sustain what is happening inside his body. Take three or four very deep breaths. Close your eyes for a few seconds. Press your hands together and promise yourself that you are going to offer everything in your power to this moment in time. Choose a sentence or phrase that you can keep repeating to yourself when you feel caught up with being afraid or in panic. "I WILL see this through . . ." or "We are going to do this together . . ." Offer a prayer to the unknown collective forces to help you both through this time.

Reassure him that you have everything under control, that you have telephoned for medical help, and ask him to try and be as still and relaxed as he possibly can be in the circumstances. Whatever has happened to the heart, it needs all the energy and oxygen it can get to sort itself out and restore some balance. There is nothing that can alter this fact. In helping him to relax and concentrate on slow breathing, you must help him to avoid hyperventilating. Often when people are afraid of having another heart attack, they overbreathe, or breathe too deeply. If he is able to take a deep breath, then three or four are enough. The more shallow breathing, faint panting, will probably be more comfortable until the initial acute pain lessens. Hyperventilation is dangerous; it leads to tingling sensations in the hands and feet, dizziness and nausea, and predisposes towards arrhythmias and coronary arterial spasm. If you realise that the patient is hyperventilating, get him to breathe into a paper bag to restore the carbon dioxide level in his blood. An injection of a pain-killing drug will help to take away some of the intense pain and will aid relaxation when medical help arrives. If your partner has been vomiting it would be unwise to give him anything to drink. Sometimes brandy has a relaxing effect but it takes time, and it also involves the work of the digestive system and the circulation and this all expends energy. By the time it takes effect medical aid might have arrived.

Do not move your patient unless absolutely necessary. If he is sitting in a chair leave him there. If he is sitting at the table having a meal, leave him where he is unless he is very uncomfortable. If he is in an upright chair it is easier for two people to lift the whole chair towards a car or ambulance. If he is already uncomfortable move him gently into a semi-prone position on the floor or on a sofa. Do not try and get him upstairs.

Loosen any clothing that might be tight and restrict

circulation, i.e. belt, tie, collar, socks, shoes, jacket.

Hold his hand, smooth his brow, talk to him softly, reassure him that he will be O.K.

IF HE LOSES CONSCIOUSNESS

If this happens you will need to apply first aid or call for someone near you who has this knowledge. It is not an easy thing to give first aid to someone close to you, but if there is no-one else you will have to. If your partner becomes unconscious you will need to make sure he can breathe properly. He needs to be on his side, with his head on one side and chin up, so that the tongue does not block his airway. The best position is the recovery position which can be learnt from any first aid course. These courses are available throughout the country from the St. John Ambulance Brigade and the British Red Cross.

If your patient stops breathing altogether you need to give mouth–to–mouth resuscitation. He must be lying on his back with you kneeling by his right side. You pull the forehead back with your left hand at the same time as pinching both nostrils together. This ensures that the airway will be as open as possible and that none of the air you are about to blow into the mouth will escape. With your right hand you open the mouth by pulling down the chin. You need to make sure that there is nothing in the mouth before you begin resuscitation, and you need to take out false teeth if there are any. To begin resuscitation you take in a good lungful of air and give four blows through your patient's mouth. You will be able to watch, from the position you are in, and see if the chest rises as you blow in air. If breathing does not commence at this point you need to resuscitate – blow in air, at a rate of about twelve per minute . . . or one every five seconds.

If the pulse rate goes and your partner's heart has stopped beating you will need to begin cardiac massage. Still kneeling at his right side, take your right arm, place your fingertips at the throat and measure the distance of three hands down to the sternum bone. Strike this place very hard with the edge of your hand. If the pulse does not return (the pulse at the jugular vein is the best one to take for this) begin cardiac massage and resuscitation. If you have someone with you you might share this work. The method is to give four blows of air into the lungs and twelve pressures onto the heart. This is achieved by placing the left hand onto the heart, palm downwards, and the right hand on top of this, also palm downwards. Then, using the weight and rhythm of your body, press twelve times, at about one per second, onto this area. Every time you finish the sequence of massage and mouth-to-mouth, check to see if the pulse has returned.

It is very difficult to learn this kind of first aid from reading a book, but it is better to have some idea than none at all, and if you only have a book to refer to in these times it is better than nothing. It is a good idea, however, for everyone to learn the rudiments of first aid at some time in their life. Even if your partner doesn't need it, someone else may. The important thing to remember in the instance of pulse failure and breathing stoppage is that there are only three to four minutes in which brain cells can live without a supply of oxygen. After this there is deterioration and brain damage. Resuscitation must begin within three minutes after breathing and pulse rate have stopped.

THE ACUTE HEART ATTACK

If your partner suddenly collapses, is immediately unconscious, and his heart and breathing have stopped, obviously first aid is vital to save his life. An ambulance should be called and first aid commenced without delay. Of the quarter of a million people who suffered heart attacks last year, of the 75,000 who died, half did so within the first two hours after the attack. First aid and prompt medical attention could possibly have saved some of these lives.

HEART ATTACKS CAN HAPPEN ANYWHERE

Many people do in fact have their heart attack at home. However, if you are on holiday, or staying with friends, you will have to rely on whatever medical facilities are available. The same principles that have been outlined will apply, but your communication skills will be very important, especially if there is another language to consider. A good thing to remember is that you are the one person who knows your partner best. Your skill and determination is needed to get him to the best medical help available, your patience and persistence might be called upon, all your charm, tolerance or even obstinacy might have to be used if you have difficulty in being understood, or paid any attention to. Having made your decision, that your partner needs medical help, you need to remember what it is you want from your communication – telephone or otherwise, with medical authorities. Try not to be fobbed off with vague answers or platitudes, but stick to what you want to get across and don't stop until you are satisfied. This may sound harsh, but it is surprising how many medical authorities can appear offhand, disinterested, and, if you sound hesitant, not quite sure, apologetic for having bothered them, downright rude and abrasive. You do not know what attitude you are going to run into if you are away from home, and it is best to act positive and sound confident and definite. A practice of the assertion technique of the broken record . . . going over the one sentence which contains what you want from the situation at stake, over and over again, sticking to it in the face of all opposition or change of subject, will help you enormously at this time. For example:

You (speaking to a foreign hospital) Please send a doctor, my husband is having a heart attack.

Hospital What are his symptoms?

You His colour is grey, he has a terrible pain in his chest, he cannot get comfortable, his arms ache, it hurts to breathe.

Hospital Has he had this before?

You Please send a doctor.

Hospital . . . Hmmm . . . you say terrible pain . . . where exactly?

You   Right across his chest, like a steel band . . . Please send a doctor.

Hospital   . . . A steel band . . .

You   Please send a doctor.

Hospital   Your name please?

You   Mrs Peter Jones, Lamare Hotel, Beach Road, Room 113. Please send a doctor.

Hospital   How old is your husband?

You   48 . . . Please send a doctor.

Hospital   Stop asking for a doctor, I'm the only one here, and I can't come out to everyone who calls.

You   This is very urgent. If you will not come out to my husband will you send an ambulance for him, or is there another doctor I could send for? I do need a doctor.

Hospital   You are quite positive that this is serious.

You   I am quite positive. Please send a doctor.

Hospital   All right then; I'll be there in ten minutes.

This example is, of course, exaggerated, to show the point about the broken record technique. By not being fobbed off with inconsequential comments like the repeat of "a steel band", or drawn into the other person's problems such as "I'm the only one here", and not being put off achieving your goal of getting a doctor to your partner, you are more likely to get a positive response than otherwise.

Receiving a message from a stranger, or from the sister of a hospital casualty department to say that your partner has suffered a heart attack is always a tremendous shock. You might feel guilty because you were not there to help him or be with him. However, these things *do* happen, you cannot be there very minute of the day, and there are plenty of other things you can do whilst he is in hospital or recovering at home. It is best to try and not worry, it is negative energy, and you will need all the positive energy you can muster for the months ahead of you. If it is helpful, use the same grounding ritual that I described under the heading *What you can do whilst waiting for the doctor or ambulance*. Be calm and relaxed. Take three or four deep breaths. Close your eyes for a few seconds. Press your hands together and promise yourself that you are going to offer everything in your power to this moment in time. Choose a sentence or phrase that will help sustain you. Light a candle and imagine your partner, wherever he is, in this circle of light, being protected by its radiance. Offer a prayer to the unknown collective forces, your God or whatever you might wish to call it.

WHAT WILL YOUR PARTNER BE FEELING?

Your partner will be suffering from shock as well as from pain. Whilst he is having the attack, whether you are alone with him or with him in hospital, the strengh of your presence will be very important to him and do not underestimate this strength. However gruff, obstinate or 'stiff upper lip' his personality may appear, the time of a heart attack is an extremely vulnerable-making, fearful and lonely occasion. The heart is a vital, potent organ. Most people know that heart disease is the main cause of death in Western countries, and many men in their middle years secretly dread it happening to them. Because heart attacks happen suddenly, the amount of shock is very great. Shock may produce silence, trembling, coldness, tears, muttering incoherently, moaning. You can respond to this with warmth rather than with fear. Support and confidence are most needed at this time. Words may be unnecessary. If breathing becomes painful it may be good to suggest that your partner breathes in short pants, from the top of his lungs, rather than take in deep breaths. Help him to 'dissociate' as described in Chapter 1.

Heart muscle is the strongest and thickest muscle in the body. When a heart attack has taken place, and heart muscle has died because a block in the coronary artery meant that no oxygenated blood supply reached it, the whole heart is thrown into chaos. The heart has to pump blood around the rest of the body, as well as pumping blood around itself, and to and from the lungs. It has an electrical system which controls and regulates the beat of the heart and the pressure between one chamber and another. After an attack, there is much work for the heart to do, but it is amazing how much potential there is for sorting itself out, restoring balance and compensating for the damage done. This work is very much assisted by the relaxation and co-operation of the rest of the body, and from an accepting, unharrassed mental attitude.

At this point, you must have faith in the work of the heart, and in your partner's capacity to recover.

Let him know that you have this faith.

Chapter 6

The Long Term View

a. *Anxiety, Fear and Guilt*

HUMAN BEINGS are alone in their experience of anxiety in our living, breathing world. Animals are said to have 'vigilance' which can last for as long as ten minutes, and all creatures experience variations of the 'startle pattern'. This response is a primary, innate, involuntary reaction which precedes the emotions of fear and anxiety. It occurs before we know what threatens us. Physically, the startle pattern manifests itself in a general flexing of the body, blinking of eyes, the head moves forward, shoulders are raised, trunk moves forward, abdomen contracts, knees bend. The startle pattern seems to be the first indication that a gap exists between the individual and his world. L. S. Kubie writes: "a foetus cannot experience startle, but the infant and his startle pattern are born at the same time". Thereafter there exists a 'gap' or 'distance' between the individual and his environment. The infant experiences waiting, postponement, frustration. Anxiety and the thought processes both arise out of this situation, with anxiety preceding the development of thought. Anxiety in the life of the individual stands as a bridge between the startle pattern and the dawn of thought. Patterns of fear and anxiety develop from this point, some more powerful in their effect than others. It would seem that anxiety is most acute when this original 'gap' is re-experienced in different ways throughout life. One of the gaps we have been talking about in this book, is the gap experienced between the ego and the self. The wider this gap, the greater the feelings of anxiety; this is coupled with feelings of alienation in life, unconnectedness, frustration, meaninglessness and frequently a deep sense of rage.

We live in an anxiety-making world, with global threat of extinction, everyday war, violence, degradation, where people in some countries are dying of famine, malnutrition, starvation, and others, not a few thousand miles away, are dying of diseases apparently induced by over-eating, affluence, too fast a living, toxic inhalation and numerous examples of excesses. Anxiety about these matters is on some level, whether conscious or not, present in us all. It could be called a natural response to an anxiety-provoking stimulus which causes us to be alert to wider concepts and to develop our thinking accordingly. Anxiety, in this context, is a healthy, intelligent, thinking person's reaction, a 'driving force' to look further. What we are concerned about in this chapter is over-anxiety, the kind of anxiety that clouds everyday living, that stops us acting with clarity rather than spurring us forward.

We all have something which makes us anxious, and many of us walk around within the fog of anxiety not always realising what it is we are enveloped in. How many people around you walk or talk very fast, in fact do everything very quickly all the time, whether eating, moving or laughing? See if you can start noticing how people sit or stand, how they hold themselves or swallow food. How many people rush into conversation without really listening to what the other person is saying, run from their car into the house or from their house up the street . . . the man who is always looking at his watch or twiddling with his cuff links? Under all of these habits is anxiety. Test your own reflexes within this framework . . . do you jump when the telephone rings? . . . do you leap about in your stomach when someone shouts in the street because you think they are shouting at you? . . . do you feel guilty when something has happened to someone else as though it must be your fault? When someone gets angry with you do you dissolve into a jelly? If you feel angry with someone do you stay silent, churning away inside, or go away and eventually decide it's you who should apologise for feeling angry? All these behaviour patterns are connected with anxiety. It can be very deeply seated and there are many psychological interpretations based on each individual experience, but this is not the function of this book. The first step towards managing everyday anxiety within ourselves is for us to become aware of it and the way in which it manifests itself, and to determine how much our lives are limited or hampered by the results of our anxiety.

When we are over-anxious, we add another pressure to our life and carry the burden unaware of it. These subtle anxieties rob us of the freedom to experience pleasure or relaxation and of our right to live openly, in love or joy or happiness. It often takes a crisis such as a heart attack for us to realise just how much anxiety is undermining our enjoyment or our participation in life, and on top of this we have the anxiety induced by the crisis itself. Firstly we need to become aware of the anxiety which is inflicted on our behaviour every day. Just take a look at what you do in a day and a closer look at the way in which you do it. Are you aware of a constant feeling of pressure, of having to push on, of feeling guilty if you relax or sit down . . . do you have to make excuses if someone calls unexpectedly and finds you reading a magazine or sipping a cup of coffee . . . do you over-justify your desire to watch football on a Saturday afternoon or to play with the dog on the lawn? Is there an overall feeling that all the time you should be getting on with duty, with chores, with a 'labelled' occupation with an 'identifiable' structure, one that is rewarded by money or status, so that without this 'order' or framework you flounder around in guilt? Can you identify yourself as having the 'A' type personality I describe in Chapter 7? . . . If these things apply to you, you are suffering from anxiety. We get anxious when we don't feel we have enough 'ego' strengths to offer life outside us, but are, at the same time, not in touch with our inner 'self'. Our uncertainty about our skills makes us anxious about presenting ourselves; our lack of belief in our own judgement makes us anxious when faced with a decision or when we are up against someone forceful or accusing. Developing a greater sense of 'wholeness', of being in touch with the two sides of our personality by shortening the gap between the two, does enable us to stand more firmly on the earth, placing ourselves in a centred position to meet life as it comes towards us.

So, what can you do with this turmoil of feelings?

Ask yourself to do a small exercise. Every time you are

conscious of feeling anxious, write it down . . . write the moment you were aware of it and what event or conversation preceded this feeling. After a few days a pattern will emerge . . . you will recognise that certain things make you feel anxious. Ask yourself' what you can do about the factors which you find anxiety-making. If there is nothing you can do, ask yourself what is the worst thing that can happen under the threat of the event with which you are concerned . . . take this to its farthest point. Having done this, ask yourself whether you could live with this or if it is as bad as you imagine. Then explore what you can do about it, or what you can offer your source of anxiety that will develop a platform from which you may begin not to be anxious. See if you can evaluate where your fears are coming from and how you can assuage them . . . this is not repression I am talking about, but an opportunity to understand your own nature in a little more depth and a call for compassion as to your own needs. See if you can ask your strengths to help your weaknesses . . . what can you put on that platform that will be of positive value to you rather than have the undermining effect of anxiety? Another question to ask is . . . do you need your anxiety? What will happen if you stop feeling anxious . . . write all this down; see what this tells you.

FOR THE PARTNER OR FAMILY OF THE HEART ATTACK PATIENT

When you find yourself getting anxious about your spouse, if they are late home, or seem depressed or can't get to sleep, just stay with the feeling you have and see if it tells you anything . . . ask the feeling what it would like you to do with it . . . what you can offer it that would be of value . . . it may be something practical like a cup of hot milk, or something soothing like a bath, something absorbing like a book, magazine or television programme. Don't start thinking that this kind of activity doesn't solve the problem, which of course it doesn't, but it might stop your anxiety escalating to the point where you are almost rigid, and the possibility of pathological change within your body tissues has set in. Being aware of anxious situations, or what is likely to lead to anxious situations, is the first step to overcoming this problem. Of course, at first, anxiety is the kind of experience that you find yourself gripped by and appears to come from nowhere. It might seem inconceivable to you that you can ever get to grips with it or do anything about it. But if you never try and understand anxiety, get a picture for it in your mind so that you have isolated something tangible with which to deal, or begin to use the strengths that you do have to combat anxiety's wringing fog, you will always be immersed in it.

Sometimes, it helps, if you are the wife of a heart attack patient, to foresee that you are going to feel anxious, to accept this, and to add it to all the things you are having to do in a day. To say "I'm going to see X today, Fred is going to be late home tonight after his dinner and I'm going to be anxious". Add it on to everything else then you won't be surprised when it happens.

The first time you find yourself in the grip of worry and anxiety connected with your husband . . . maybe the first time he goes out in the car, or stays late in the office, gets drunk, or wants to do something he's been told not to do, see if you can go along with it, accepting the anxiety. At the same time you can ask yourself what you can do about the situation that is happening. Can you stop him doing any of the things you get anxious about? If he were to stop would this make any difference? How do you feel about stopping him do something because of your anxiety? Might your anxiety make him feel more anxious and leave the two of you in a puddle of anxiety and worry, never able to get out of it? If you can't stop him doing something, but have to learn to accept this aspect of his behaviour just as you accept the way in which he cleans his teeth or reads the newspaper, you are left with your anxiety and it falls back on you to suffer through it until you are able to handle it more comfortably. None of us ever stops feeling anxious at times; anxiety is the normal reaction of a sensitive person to something difficult or fearsome. It's *over-anxiety* you need to watch for and sort out. Another useful idea is to make sure you have facts to go on . . . that you know where he is going and might be contacted, although you would never use this information. The unknown is the most worrying factor of all in these matters because then you are left with the depths of your imagination. Time, too, is useful. Set a loose deadline . . . "if he doesn't come by midnight" . . . "eight o'clock", whatever, "then

I will have a think and a cup of tea . . . if it gets to nine o'clock I will ring up a friend and talk to her" . . . and so on. Plan your time and try not to keep looking at the clock or standing at a window waiting to hear the sound of a car or taxi or key in the lock of the front door. These kinds of activities only serve to inflame your already existing anxiety further. Remember, too, that buses *are* often late, people may keep him talking late, and he may simply have met someone he hasn't seen for years and gone for a pint!

When your husband feels anxious and it's obvious that worry is making him tense and restless, you need then to put yourself in a position of strength and place your own anxieties on one side. It is not always easy to do because your own anxieties are so wrapped up with his. But practice helps, and so does trying to put yourself into the position of being your partner. Imagine that it is you who has had the heart attack. How would you feel, what are your fears, what is it like from your body? See what pictures you get from doing this and see whether it offers you any enlightenment, any help or understanding. Then you are in a position of greater strength to help your husband than if you are within the wobbly part of your own need. Feel out to him as much as you can, and try and premeditate things that are going to be difficult. Women are in a particularly good position to take some of the strain off a man because of the way in which they operate. Women often have a capacity for a broader thinking base, a diffuse, rather than focused, outlook. But the greatest help of all is for you to learn to deal with your own anxieties not pass them on to him. Your quiet confidence and determination is the greatest reassurance and 'back up' he can have, and can foil many of his worries at source.

b.   Confidence – Yours and your Family's

It often happens that people lose confidence after a major illness. They have to start again in so many fundamental areas at the same time as carrying the burden of their own expectations which have grown with their years of living. A heart attack brings many emotions to the surface, and so does lying helpless in bed. Tears can quickly be drawn and this can make you feel you are losing your grip, not the man or woman you were. There is nothing like getting on and doing things to stimulate confidence and this, regardless of the ups and downs, is the only way it will be regained after a heart attack. The first areas concern your health and stamina because this is where you will feel a loss of confidence the most at first. In having to do things slowly, little by little, you might find you have to cope with a busy, impatient mind which will try and force you to hurry, to move on and to judge your performance, telling you you're not good enough. Try and put your impatient mind on one side, 'on ice' if you like, for the time being, and concentrate on just exactly what you are able to do at one given moment in time.

In building up confidence that has been lost or never been claimed, we need to begin in a small way. Being confident about yourself when you look in the mirror is a start. Have a look at what you see . . . are you on friendly terms with the figure before you, or do you give the person you see a hard time? What are your expectations of that person . . . what do you ask of them, how much do you try and push them through in a day . . .how many of the things that you do are you doing because you really want to, and how many because of duty, habit or someone else told you to? Make a list under each heading. Think of the things you do well and ask yourself why you do them well, what is the motivation behind them, why is it that doing those particular tasks allows you to have no thought about confidence, or lack of it? (The idea is to establish for yourself the reality of your own natural energy source.) What is confidence, anyway? How do you see it? What do you see as confidence in someone else . . . is it a quality that you admire? Set about thinking what you mean by confidence. For me, confidence is going into an experience from a 'centre' that does not oscillate or teeter from one side to another. It is having that calm assuredness that is not dependent on the opinions of others.

So many of us get pressured into doing things at times when we are too young to question them and find ourselves still doing them and responding to old and out-of-date stimuli long after they have ceased to be relevant in our lives. Even guilt can be a habit, based on "mother wouldn't like it" or "better not let Dad see me enjoying myself", or whatever. When we are adult, we can choose whether or not we want to go on living with these kinds of responses. But we need to recognise what we are doing first.

If you are the husband, wife or relative of the patient reading this, it is likely that your confidence will be rocked more severely by your partner's moods than their health. You have possibly been through an illness yourself, or maybe you have given birth to children. If you are the wife of the patient, perhaps you have had to deal with your own slowness and gradual return to busy life and the fluctuation of your own moods after the birth of children or during the adjustment period being at home after working full-time. There is nothing as fragmentary as being a housewife and mother of young children at home all day, and it is an excellent training ground for the understanding of moods. Many men never have to go through this experience, and when they do it scares them rigid. But you, as a woman, if you know what I am talking about, will be able to be sympathetic and helpful. That very patience you learned the hard way will help you to recognise what is superficial in the displays of tempestuousness and frustration from your partner, and to react accordingly. You can learn when not to take these moods too seriously, and certainly, *never* personally. As the wife of a heart attack patient, you must recognise hurt pride, personal frustration, difficulties and disappointments within himself that he doesn't even want to share with you, so gets cross and moody instead. Confront the mood as a symbol of the recovery process and not as a reflection on your personality. Lighten the atmosphere where possible, don't let it get heavy. Your understanding will give him something to go on, something to test himself out against. You can become the barometer against whom he measures himself for stabilisation . . . and for a good laugh. This testing out may not end here but may go on to also test *you* out . . . *your* loyalty, *your* endurance, *your* love. This is hard, but it happens.

c.   Handling Defeat

We feel defeated when our ambitions are not reached, our hopes not realised, our goals seem far away, and when we can no longer inspire hope in ourselves. These goals and ambitions may be of the everyday kind – coping well with children, with parking the car, not eating too much, finding the right gift for a friend. Or they might be something larger and more continuous – succeeding at work, finding a good relationship, overcoming a particular fear.

The feeling of defeat seems to come after a series of disappointments. Often we can shrug off the first few disappointments and not worry unduly about the odd failure, telling ourselves that we can't have everything and to just keep on trying. We energise ourselves to start again, pick ourselves up and have another go. But when we have to deal with what we see as repeated disappointment and failure, our sense of personal worth and self confidence becomes under more severe strain as we struggle to do more and more to overcome what we believe are our shortcomings.

There may be many things which we consider to be against us – a poor support system at home or in terms of educational background – we may feel we have to work harder than others to counteract a slow start, a weak memory, or skills we don't feel we have grasped well enough. We may also have many personal worries about money, housing, children, older and dependent relations. Sometimes we even attempt to take on the government or the entire social services department in order to vent our rage at what we feel is unfair, or against us.

There is a point at which our feelings of defeat are accompanied by enormous frustration – fury at being stuck inside something we consider immoveable – and we struggle furiously to try to gain control of what can become an ever increasing nightmare. If this situation continues we eventually reach a breakdown in health. Homeostatis is violated and we lose resistance to illness. Later our rage may turn to feelings of despair, hopelessness, defeat and distress. When these 2 patterns carry on for some time our bodies experience an increase of the arousal of the sympatho-adrenomedullary system which invokes increased catecholamine secretion. Associated with the feelings of despair and defeat is high pituitary-adreno-cortical arousal. The arousal of these hormones known as S-AM and P-AC can occur simultaneously, and their activities are highly catabolic. They "mobilise all the mechanisms that produce energy for coping, and suppress the mechanisms that store energy or use it for growth, repair and surveillance against pathogens. As part of this adaptive response the brain mobilises cardiac, vascular and renal mechanisms to raise the blood pressure. When arousal is chronic, the high pressure causes damage which, in interaction with a variety of arousal induced chemical changes, leads to end-stage diseases such as stroke and kidney disease and coronary heart disease."* Our attitude to our work and daily lives affects not only our emotional and psychological life, but also the chemistry of our bodies and if we are off-balance in the way just described then we give our bodies the wrong and inappropriate messages.

If we realise that we have a repeated pattern of disappointment, or failing at something, no matter how hard we work or how long we struggle, it is a good idea to examine on what basis it is that we have rested our desires, our motivation and our expectations. Rather than carry on struggling, we need to ask ourselves what we are doing wrong. We need to be able to take a step back and look at how we do things rather than push blindly on under the umbrella of overwork, hoping that this will cure all. It may not. We need to start by examining our premises and to do this we need to remove ourselves from the treadmill existence where we struggle against the fear of defeat, even if only for a few days. Talking to someone else about what we are doing may help, someone who will help us to see our situation objectively. We need to assess our skills, talents, personality, tastes, hopes. We need to return in some way to basics, to examine what it is we work for, struggle for, what our priorities are. Then we need to ask: are these struggles, priorities, goals, appropriate to my needs, my skills, my

* *The Practitioner*, September 1982. Dr. P.G.F. Nixon FRCP.

lifestyle? We may long to be a movie star, a tycoon who earns lots of money or a racing driver . . . but have we kept this dream on a dream level, or have we tried, perhaps unrealistical-ly, to make them become the reality of our lives? Are we ruled by them, rather than enjoying them as fantasy? Do we hear someone else's voice urging us on with a task that if we were to look at it realistically we are unsuited to? Maybe that voice is a powerful one, so loud in our ears that the minute it utters we mobilise all our energies and adrenalin and get into racing speed automatically. We need to face these, our demons, before they rule us and run us into the ground. Once named and placed appropriately within our being they are much easier to deal with. "Be quiet Nick" you can say as you feel that wicked voice nudging you bullyingly into overdrive and overwork.

If we look at dreams more realistically we need to go back and remember what our original dreams once were. Often these are the seedbed of what is right for us. They contain some original ideas about ourselves that can become obscured by the training and programming of our families and schools. Or it may have been simply unrealistic to take up such dreams before. Now life is asking us to do so.

So far we have been looking towards assessing our life and its current difficulties and asking if we are in the right place. If, after assessment, we decide that we are, or that we cannot change anything, we need to examine what exactly it is that makes us feel defeated. If we feel defeated because we feel that life is against us we need to reappraise on what basis that should be. What puts life or people against us? Do we presume that because people are not obviously *for* us they are therefore *against* us? Do we defeat ourselves with our own attitude? Do we feel defeated because we are always comparing ourselves with other people and always finding someone who is better, fitter, bigger, stronger, happier, more glamorous, successful than we are? If this is our way we will always feel defeated because we will always find someone who will fit into this pattern of being better than we are. Have we set our goals too high? Are they realistic? If our goals are inappropriately high and we have no stepping stone method of getting to one small goal at a time then we will always feel defeated.

Handling defeat is reappraising what it is that makes us feel defeated and placing it properly within the context of our lives. Nevertheless there will be times when we have tried and tried at something and it has just not worked out. We may know with hindsight that we were aiming high. Maybe we married the wrong man or woman because we hoped they would spread a little of their warmth, humour, or whatever, in our direction so that we wouldn't have to work quite so hard at developing our own. We may realise that we have bitten off more than we can chew. But this does not help those terrible feelings of defeat that we all have to contend with at some point. We need a time away to heal those wounds, replenish energies that have been spent out and to begin to think and emerge again.

It is important to believe that it is not 'me', the person, who is defeated but the aspect of the behaviour that drove us onto the particular path that appears to have ended in disaster. There are some feelings of defeat that have nothing to do with our own effort and many of us have to find the bravest and most philosophical ways we can of living with them; for example the defeat we may feel when someone we love is ill or disabled and we reach out to them in their struggle to find a way to cope with the details of simple living. We may feel defeated with politicians at the arrival of Cruise missiles in Britain despite large and impressive protests, we may feel defeated by the ravages of war, the apparent unfairness of loss, the inevitability of the elements and the passing of time. Unless we can actively crusade against these things we must actively crusade against their intrusion by way of feelings of despair and defeat into the fabric and chemistry of our minds and bodies.

If we have the energy and conviction to fight against what we believe to be evil or for something we much believe in, then we must let that take us where it will and acknowledge that defeat may be part of that journey we choose to make. Some people never acknowledge defeat but carry on mobilising their strengths which would seem to come from the passion of their feelings. If we think positively we are not defeated and we are still getting a great deal out of what we are struggling for. But when the smell of defeat invades us and begins to weigh us down, we must stop and consider whether or not we are on the right path.

If we stay in touch with ourselves and our needs, pay respect to our being as a whole, know what motivates and energises us healthily and creatively, we can stay on top of our defeats, accepting them as part of life, mourning a little for the loss they create, and then move on.

d. For Wives and Partners: Responsibility, Nursing and Old Wives' Tales

In all probability you have so far acted as nurse and handmaiden . . . a rôle which many of us find comes very easily and we welcome it, but if you're not careful it can become a trap.

If you have felt that, at last, what a chance to be really needed . . . to have a clear place at your partner's side, to be important to him again at a time when you might have been questioning this . . . you might be tempted to supercharge yourself up to a great pitch of self-importance and, in the process, swamp the results of the grand effort you are making. For example . . . if your partner needs to have medication, in the beginning it is a good idea to share this responsibility with him, especially if he is unused to taking pills, and to ask if he has had his twelve o'clock pills or his four o'clock pills, or whatever. It is also a good idea to see in advance if he is likely to run out and to organise a new supply or prescription if appropriate. The same thing goes with the amount of sleep, exercise, social commitments, work. In the beginning it is all new ground for you both and you need to share the testing out of his strength and your resolve not to be anxious. His pacing himself with you knowing quietly what he is doing is quite different from the order and precision he has received in hospital. It is a mistake to try and emulate that . . . to become bossy and sharp, to work everything by the letter like a regimental march. Convalescing is very much a learning process . . . it is time and space to discover what is comfortable and what is not, what needs looking at and what does not, what is important, what is not. It is a very fundamental time for you both and it needs an elastic tolerance. If you find that you are becoming rather aggressive about when and how often he takes his exercise or sticks to his routine ask yourself who you are doing it for . . . for him or yourself? See if it isn't some underlying anxiety of your own that isn't coming out on the surface as aggression and rigidity, or maybe there is some unexpressed anger. If you need to look at this read the next section on this subject.

So, back to this particular subject, responsibility. It's *his* heart attack and an important part of his becoming well is for him to accept the responsibility not only for having the disease in the first place, but also for recovering from it and making sure that it doesn't happen again. When the emergency has passed, your rôle as nurse needs to pack itself neatly away in its Mary Poppins bag and the you as woman, partner, lover, mistress, helpmate, friend, confidant, admirer and playmate needs to come to the forefront, and the experience you have both been through together will have had the opportunity of developing this. If you stay with the rôle of nurse too long you will rob your man of his masculinity. You will encourage him to be kept as a child and his rages will have the unreason and ferocity of a four year old's. His frustration will be immense. In slowly weaning off his dependence on you as a nurse you are handing over to him the reins of his own life and his own body. There is a point where your work in this sense is over . . . you may keep a watchful eye from a distance, but keep it to yourself, and recognise that much of the energy you put into it is for your own peace of mind. It is hard to let go, to take the risk of his forgetting, or running out of pills on a Friday night when there is no surgery until Monday morning, of swimming too hard that he has indigestion for the rest of the day, or getting so drunk that he doesn't know what is happening to him. But your letting go is the only way he is going to know his limitations and the only way he can learn how to deal with his own needs. If you are always there to do it for him he will never move on, he will be denied the privilege of exploring himself, of finding out the result of his own private little tests on himself and his strength. If you've had children, think back to the time when your son and daughter caught the bus back from school for the first time; not the one you had mapped out for them, but another one because it was quicker or it came first, even though it put them off at a different place to where you had shown them it would; and you realised that a bit of their own individuality had emerged for the first time, a bit of survival mechanism, something that no-one can take away from them; a priceless acknowledgement. It is wicked to rob anyone of this small claim to independence and growth and the same applies to your partner's taking responsibility for his own illness.

It doesn't mean that you don't care, simply that you are not carrying it all for him but giving him the opportunity to find out for himself. There are ways of pointing out that he has been overdoing it, or is looking rather tired or that the garden doesn't need digging over again. One of the ways is to organise your life together wherever you can so that he is free from stress or overwork and has enough space in which to continue with his own rehabilitation. Make sure that you don't have too many visitors one after the other . . . don't ask him if he wants them or can manage . . . just allow the space so that he doesn't have to make a decision of that kind. If it is possible, organise time away together as often as you can or time when he can develop hobbies or interests that other commitments have crowded out. Let him see that you are busy too, are getting on with your life so that he doesn't have to worry about you. If you are not hurrying or anxious or fretful or depressed then he is less likely to be. All you can do to lessen these burdens on your life will be helpful to you both.

You will find that people will bombard you with good advice and their own brand of old wives' tales. If you are unsure (as inevitably we all *are* at such a time) and possibly eager for advice or other opinions, then the comments of friends will make a strong impression on you. This has its good and bad points. It's not good to be pulled from one extreme to another because you get off-centre at a time when you need to be sticking to one point of view, and too many other views can be very confusing.

Everyone has their own particular fetish or bit of specialist knowledge that they feel qualified to pass on to another. Everyone has their own pet remedy, cure, doctor, book, story to illustrate the rightness of what they are saying, and are convinced that if only you will take up with their ideas all will be well. This just isn't so. Everyone is different and responds differently to cures and pills. What you are struggling to find is the way that suits your partner and yourself and the only way towards this aim is by sticking to what suits you. All advice and remarks are intended to be helpful and often can be, but just as often they may not be. The worst kind of remarks are those which insinuate that you are in some way responsible for your partner's recovery and that you have sole control in what he does. Remarks such as "You're not letting him ride his motorbike, are you?" or "I hope you're not giving him butter/cooking with animal fat anymore" or "you should be making him stick to a light diet", "you mustn't let Bob go down to the pub on his own", "you don't mean to tell me that you've approved of his carrying on smoking" are downright hurtful as well as unhelpful and are guaranteed to make you feel inadequate and to rub salt into your already present wound. As if you could stop him raiding the cake tin in the middle of the night or racing off on his motorbike before you got the car out, and don't these people think you would give your eye teeth for him to stop smoking . . . ? What's it got to do with them anyway, why don't they mind their own business and stop wasting your energy!!

There are so many myths about what happens to your life's partnership when one of you has a heart attack. People eyed me with pity when they said "Of course I suppose it's all over for you now in the bedroom department" or "I suppose you can't expect him to climb up all those stairs anymore and will have to move house" or "you won't want to come to the parties at Christmas now with Fred having his bad heart".

It's almost as though there are people around who might rejoice in their partner's descent into dependence, or as though they relish the thought of your life having to accommodate the unthinkable. A heart attack certainly changes your life but it by

THE HEART ATTACK RECOVERY BOOK

no means diminishes it. Rather the opposite: it allows you a breathing space from the pace of life to have a look at what is important and to concentrate on this, making it better, not writing it off and both sex and parties may be better than ever before. Having a bad heart is an expression used so glibly by people and conjures up an image of a weak person, barely able to hobble about on two legs, needing permanent access to an oxygen bottle and who might go out like a light at any minute, if you so much as squeeze them or speak too loud, let alone wrap your arms around them in a warm embrace or suggest a romp in the swimming bath. It's time such illusions were shattered. There *are* unfortunate people who are very ill with heart conditions and who do need special care and attention, but for the majority of heart attack patients there is overwhelming evidence around of a return to working and playing life in the fullness of expression. As I've said before, coping with a heart attack is a private matter between your partner and yourself and those whom you choose to include. Try and keep it that way.

e. *Anger*

We haven't really said enough about anger.

Anger is such a taboo subject in the Western world although we see displays of it and read about them every day in the newspapers and all about us. In a time of rising unemployment and economic recession there is always a climate of anger which bursts its way out of conventional bounds in hooliganism, vandalism, increase in violent crime and muggings, in over-spending, overeating and other acts of self-punishment.

Most of us find it very difficult to express anger and often only realise how angry we are when a sharp remark escapes from our lips or we lose our tempers with the car when it won't start or with the girl in the bank who is slow giving us our money. Often we think of what we should have said after the appropriate time and are even more angry with ourselves for not having stood up for ourselves in the moment. If we have angry feelings we wait until they have built up before we explode with them rather than acknowledge them as we go along. Often we don't know what to do with anger and we let the moment pass and the anger is dispersed somewhere in our bodies, never having been expressed. In every life crisis there is always anger. "Why me?" "Why us?" "What have I done?" "Why now?" Even if these expressions are not voiced, you may feel angry with your body for letting you down. You may not know how to deal with this, being in such a vulnerable position, and take it out on the nearest person to you. Your spouse may become the focal point for your anger because you don't know how to accept it within yourself. They may have to carry this anger for you for a period of time but there is equally a time when he or she should fight back, say "I've had enough, I'm angry too" and hand it back to you to deal with yourself.

Being angry with someone is in fact a compliment . . . you are saying . . . "what you do this minute makes me angry and I love you enough, regard you enough, to tell you so, that it may be put right between us and our relationship improved". Receiving anger is just as difficult as expressing it and often we feel totally annihilated because someone is angry with us; we feel that it is ME the person is angry with and not merely our behaviour at that time. In fact the other person is regarding us with enough trust and adulthood to be able to express him or her self in this way.

In the recovery period after illness it is important to acknowledge your angry feelings to yourself, even if you feel it inappropriate to express them outwardly. There are several things you can do to release anger by yourself and it is worth thinking about these instead of rushing to the bread and butter, making an angry 'phone call or taking out your anger on children or the dog, who cannot answer you back.

The next time that you realise you are angry try and focus on the feelings that you have. Where are the angry feelings located in the body? If you could carry the anger forward, what avenue would it take? For example would you like to punch someone in the nose, scratch their eyes out, bash their teeth in, wring their necks, throw a brick through the window, pound the butter in front of you to a pulp? Do you see red? Does your heart thump loudly in your ears, your jaw get fixed, your fists and neck tense, your stomach churn? Do you feel you could blow something up, set fire to the cause of your fury, tear it apart? All these actions are our basic instinctual response to the stress of anger. On a very primitive level they were responsible for our survival before the development of civilisation. Because they are an integral part of our make-up they appear before us and contradict the civilised social ethic we are taught is sacred to our present behaviour as a race. A civilised world does not tolerate the expression of anger. Most of us tend to avoid the expression when we can and to move away from confrontation if we see it coming. We take the indirect route, not owning up to angry feelings, but swallowing them, muttering under our breath and feeling a burning resentment later on.

Once we accept that anger is available and present, inevitable in our daily lives, what can we do with it?

Go back to the feelings of anger that you have and the outlet that your feelings tell you you might like to use. Then go and find a harmless object to use to vent your anger upon. It may be a cushion that you hurl against the wall, a towel you wring tighter and tighter in your hands, a pillow that you pound with your fists or jump upon, the earth in the garden that you stab with the old kitchen knife. You take the feelings your body so badly wants to express into an area where it is safe to do so, where no-one will get hurt but where you will have an opportunity to express yourself instead of forcing the adrenalin produced by anger back into your body. As you do any of these actions, try and vocalise your angry feelings . . . it is not easy to do at first, but to shout out words, any words . . . "damn, blast, hell . . . bugger all rules, men, children, newspapers, mothers, cakes that won't rise, cats that aren't housetrained, buses that don't run on time" . . . vent your angry feelings rightly upon the thing which produced them in the first place . . . give them some focus, let them out in a run of voiced expression. It is a great release, and you may wind up laughing at yourself and rolling on the floor afterwards. But you will no longer have the angry feelings trapped inside you, doing mischief to your physical body. These exercises will not take away the cause of your anger and frustration . . . that is something to think about when you have dealt with the anger that you are unable to put elsewhere.

What happens if you know you are angry but cannot express it? You know that it is burning away like a hot fire inside you but you cannot reach it and fear its explosive nature too much to express it. This can make us feel frustrated and helpless. Just consciously realising that you are angry is a start, and staying with the feelings that you have, letting yourself go with them when possible rather than pushing them away can be enough to help you at first. Many people are helped by Zen studies, with subjects such as anger. If you are angry, then that is the feeling you have, that is where you are, and you do the next thing that comes in the order of things. You pick up the threads of your life one at a time. If the next thread is washing the floor, that is what you do; if it is getting up from your chair, stroking the cat, bending to tie up a shoelace, this is what you do, and so on.

DISABLING ANGER

Anger is described as disabling when it cannot be reached or acknowledged, and it is often anger which began a long time ago. An individual who is angry, has a raised adrenalin level and raised blood pressure. You may notice their anger in their faces, the way they walk, the edge to their voice or the loud, clipped way in which they speak; or, they may be silently angry, creating a hostile atmosphere by the quality of their silences, the shrug of their shoulders or by grunts or huffs. Since our culture is predominantly Christian, many people take up a stoic and saintly resignation to things that actually make them very angry inside. The attitude – "one must make a sacrifice for the sake of others" – can mask unexpressed anger towards the others for whom these sacrifices are being made. This can become so fixed that even when what's going on underneath is recognised and challenged, the feelings of anger are denied in a spate of righteous indignation. It is indeed very difficult to be able to acknowledge the anger that has been thundering under the mask for years. Anger is a defence mechanism . . . it is saying: don't treat me like that, don't hurt me, if you do that again I'll ...; it is saying 'no' very loudly, and proclaiming a boundary for the self. When we decide not to express it because we think people won't love us, like us, talk to us again or won't hear us, we take up another defence mechanism, a mask, so that people won't see what we really feel and carry out all the things we dread inside that they will. The mask sends out other signals to put people off the real issue, anger. The mask says: I'm here to please you ... to make sacrifices ... I don't really matter ... one should and one ought ... for God, for one's country, for the parish, the charity, for a good cause, for the sake of the children – and after a while the mask gets believed and taken up, and people find themselves doing all sorts of things they really resent or loathe, but they are caught in this trap of masking what they really felt a long time ago. At some point along the way, this unresolved, unexpressed anger gets into the body. John Harrison writes:

If a person fails to resolve his anger, he will alter his external appearance. The internal consequences of unresolved anger are chronic elevation of blood pressure (hypertension) and shut down of the blood vessels of the hands and feet (peripheral vascular disease). All systems and organs of the body are affected by one's psychological state. After a period, they may subtly adjust to the internal milieu of their hosts, thereby passing components of the parents' psychological state to the children. Anger thus becomes inherited.*

Letting down the mask may be a painful process, but it may need to be done to release the anger that is maintaining an unhealthy arousal (stress) level throughout our body systems ... particularly the heart. Realising the long ago pattern, releasing some of the long ago resentment, however silly and long ago it may seem, can give relief to what the body is being forced to carry. The most difficult anger to deal with here is the anger associated with humiliation, defeat, impotence and a sense of helplessness, but being able to speak about it. to get in touch with what it really feels like, is the first step to positive action, away from the helpless/hopeless dichotomy. We may not be able to change our current situation externally, but we can make concessions to what

* *Love Your Disease*, John Harrison, Angus & Robertson, 1984.

we feel about it and decide then what we want to do about our resentment, fury or anger. I know someone who was burying herself up inside with anger and resentment towards her husband who, she felt, had never loved her or shown affection. In her struggle to try and 'make' him change after years of turning the other cheek, she got herself into a furious, frustrated state and pushed up her blood pressure. Only when she could acknowledge all her resentment and anger to him and the anger at herself for putting up with an unreasonable situation, could she let it go – she ritualistically burnt all her pent-up feelings by having a bonfire of all her open letters (unsent) to him. Once the burden was gone and the pressure off both of them, they could get on with their lives and she could be relieved of her raised blood pressure.

Chapter 7

Who has a Heart Attack? . . .
Some of the Theories

TRACKING DOWN the 'unknown murderer' called heart disease
has become something of a frantic and personal crusade for
medical scientists. When my interest in this subject began it
seemed to me that there was a kind of perversity in the fact that
scientists, with their broad spectrum antibiotics, have stamped
out many of the pernicious diseases such as tuberculosis,
smallpox, diptheria, that used to cream off people in their prime
of life, but are now faced with another kind of epidemic disease
which can manifest itself suddenly and without warning, when
it is too late for many of the developed wonders of science and
technology. I have an image of frustrated scientists eager to
produce new theories that might get to the bottom of this killer
disease in the simplistic way that offering a large dose of
penicillin to an infection to wipe it out has changed the face of
medicine. There is a desperation in the way the public also
rushes to absorb new theories about heart disease the minute
they take up even one column inch in the newspapers.
Commercial companies, too, play a large part in this, often
promoting research programmes and surveys. It is as if we all
seek to have something tangible to get hold of, so that we can
say "ah, yes . . . this is it . . ." and adapt ourselves accordingly.
  The risk factors that contribute to heart disease are well
enough known – smoking, too much saturated fat in the diet,
hypertension, overweight, 'A'-type personality and the hereditary factors leading to susceptibility to heart disease. But still the
most unlikely people have heart attacks, sometimes after they
have been pronounced medically fit. In the United States the
evaluation of risk factors and their being taken 'to heart' would

seem to have contributed to the fall in premature heart attack
and deaths from heart attack. In Britain, however, the numbers
continue to rise above the statistics for 1976. In that year the
death rates from coronary disease per 100,000 population aged
between 55 and 64 years were 2,394 men and 544 women in
Great Britain.

Let us look, then, at some of the theories.

a.   Risk Factors

There are avoidable and unavoidable risk factors involved in the
lives of people who become sufferers of heart attacks.

The unavoidable risk factors are age, sex, race and ethnic origin,
family history and early environment. More men than women
tend to have heart attacks in the age range under 55. From this
age on the proportion of women suffering from heart attacks
increases and in recent years the number of younger women
suffering has increased.

Britain, in particular Scotland, and Finland are the countries
which suffer the highest number of heart attacks per population. If you live in these countries you are more at risk than in
others. The Western countries have by far the greater incidence
of coronaries and the risk of the individual is greater than if he
or she lived in China or India.

There is slightly more risk of your having a coronary if there
is evidence of coronary disease running through the family, but
this may be more to do with the inheritance of other habits
which tend to point to heart attack rather than a genetically
preordained structure. Studies of diseases within the social
environment show that a deprived early life with little parental
attention, constantly shifting of home, poor eating and sleeping
habits, tend to make people much more prone to all diseases,
particularly psychiatric disease such as schizophrenia. There is
also evidence to show that the tensions, lack of confidence and
sense of personal identity stemming from a poor early start in
life, cause a prolonged, deeply held, internal stress level which

can result in the development of coronary disease, and also long depressions which can lead to suicide.

The avoidable risk factors are the most well known and documented ones and were produced after long studies in America. After the publication of the Framingham Studies in Massachusetts, many health-conscious Americans stopped smoking, started eating less animal fat, began keep-fit program-mes to strengthen their muscles and improve circulation, and watched their weight more carefully. The incidence of heart attack did fall and has continued to do so, very slightly, ever since. Heart disease still, however, remains the main cause of death in America. In Britain too, 400 people die from heart disease every day, the major cause being heart attack or myocardial infarction. In 1979, of the 90,428 people who suffered acute myocardial infarction in Britain (63,680 men and 30,600 women), 14,330 men and 10,500 women died.

The risk factors which are not so well documented and are still hotly debated in many medical circles are the risk factors of stress, tension, 'A' type personality, addiction to overwork, the attempt to overcome exhaustion and arousal with more and more work, and the devastating effect of the smell of defeat when performance does not live up to the amount of effort.

The heart's main function is to provide for effort. When this is overused, abused, overstretched, either by addiction to work and adrenalin or by the inability to deal with an overarousal of the emotions in the face of difficulty, the heart goes gradually into malfunction, sometimes taking a long time to show symptoms which can point the way to change and recovery. In their paper on acute myocardial infarction, Van Heijningen and Treurniet write: "many patients tell us that they consciously had only one wish: to grow up and become independent as quickly as possible, so as to get rid of the position of being poor, having to ask, wait one's turn, etc. And the only way to become independent is to work and work." And "coronary patients never give in. The command to be 'normal', competent and firm, and the command to pull oneself together in all circumstances, to maintain self control and leadership; in short to be 'superadapted' are so intensely cathected and rigidly represented in the superego that a hysterical solution to the conflict is out of the question. The result is a complete denial of every kind of dependence."*

Victorian physicians paid close attention to the effects of prolonged and excessive coping effort. Their natural remedy for the cardiovascular consequences of exhaustion such as hypertension, angina pectoris, vasomotor instability which lead ultimately to hyperventilation, hyperuricaemia, hyperglycaemia and fluid retention and breakdown due to the demands which outstrip the competence of the coronary circulation, was a resting, sleeping regimen followed by relaxing in comfortable circumstances and then training for a successful return to the business of living and making a living. If the above symptoms are ignored, or attempts made to try and overcome them with more work, too many drugs or cups of coffee, the progression through ill-health is toward total breakdown. In sudden cardiac death there is "a catastrophic collapse of homeostatis and loss of ability to keep the internal milieu within the limits required for survival: the trigger commonly appears to be hyperventilation-induced coronary arterial spasm or arrhythmia".†

One can only wonder and guess at how much the figures for heart attack would be changed if the above risk factors were better recognised by doctors, teachers, and society itself. A deeply held sense of work ethic which leads to overwork and overarousal instead of the successes desired, coupled with a reluctance to express one's feelings of anxiety, loss, sadness, sense of failure and struggle when this is occurring, would seem to be common generally among the Western societies, and a specific individual struggle for the coronary-prone patient. These can be changed, attitudes discussed and behaviour trained to extract more from life than being driven disastrously towards a loss of resistance to illness, and catastrophe.

* *Psychodynamic Factors in Acute Myocardial Infarction.* H. Kits Van Heijningen and N. Treurniet, Amsterdam (1965).
† *Coping, effort and the heart*, Dr. P.G.F. Nixon F.R.C.P. *New Directions in Cardiology.*

There may be another factor related specifically to men. Whereas women live in constant touch with their bodies through their monthly cycles and childbearing activities, men have no such regular involvement. Women's activities, through their bodies, give them the opportunity of being more grounded and more able to know what they are feeling and express it. This has also become more traditionally the feminine way. Since the 50's men have begun to give up their strictly macho image and allow themselves to become more feeling and more expressive, but this has occurred mostly through the initiation of women. As women became more independent they required their menfolk to be more sensitive, to be more in touch with their feelings, more gentle and soft. For many men this was a relief; now they too could begin to express their feminine side, play a little, share in household tasks, stay at home sometimes. But it would seem that there is a further step to take, to do with the male mode of feelings and discovering what this is. Robert Bly* talks about the male need to make contact with the 'wildman' at the bottom of his psyche, a step that the 70's and 80's male has not yet taken. The 'wildman', Bly believes, lies deep in the masculine energy of the psyche and relates to the very ancient, primitive instinctual forces within man that have not been initiated for a long time. The reasons for a man's grief and sense of purposelessness are often to do with a lack of wholeness, and the golden ball of wholeness lies not in men capturing feminine qualities of instinct, feeling and passion, but by seeking out their own and initiating other men along this path. This male energy is not the superficially macho or destructive and aggressive energy, but creative, powerful and deeply spiritual. A possible 'risk factor', therefore, is a certain emotional impoverishment in men who are not in touch with these more powerful feelings that give a sense of wholeness and a sense of purpose in life. When men (or women) are 'cut off' from this important source of energy, their tensions are inner dynamic ones. As yet we have little information to prove that this internal emotional arousal level is a contributory

* *What Men Really Want*, Robert Bly, New Age Magazine, USA, (May 1982).

factor in heart attack, but my subjective view is that it is in this area that most research is needed.

b. Smoking

The link between smoking and lung cancer has been firmly established in our understanding, but the links between smoking and heart disease are not as yet so widely accepted. In 1978 the Department of Health estimated that the deaths of about a quarter of the 92,367 men and 68,077 women who died of coronary heart disease were caused by smoking. Over 37,000 of the people who died were under 65. Given these statistics, we may calculate that at least 19,000 people died prematurely, whilst still of working age, because they smoked cigarettes.

This will be disheartening news to you if you smoke more than twenty cigarettes a day and have done so for a long time. If we smoke cigarettes the chances of getting a serious disease are far greater than if we don't smoke, and most of us know this but feel that we've got to die sometime so why bother. But, if you are reading this book, think on in terms of your choices in life and in terms of the quality of life that you know you have the opportunity to seek out. Do you really want to burn your way to chronic bronchitis and emphysema, chronic sinusitis, cancer of the lung, oral cavity, larynx, pharynx or bladder? The list goes on and on of diseases scientifically proven to be directly linked with smoking. Now you might say, "old Dad's smoked for years and never had a days illness" or you might be able to list scores of people who smoked like chimneys all their lives and died at ninety after being struck by a bus. This is fine. But it is only one half of it. There are equally strongly supported stories in opposition to this rather jovial view, depending on which you feel like following at the time. If you are close to someone who has already suffered from a heart attack it is worth seriously considering what the scientific studies of cigarette smoking and health have actually proved. It might just give you that extra determination you need to stop.

Nicotine increases the work of the heart whilst carbon

monoxide (present in cigarette smoke) reduces the supply of oxygen to the heart and can lead to atheroma (deposits of fatty substances in the arterial walls). Smokers of 40 cigarettes a day or more have 4 times as much atheroma as non smokers. Both nicotine and carbon monoxide increase the tendency to develop thrombosis (blood clots). Carbon monoxide, one of the most poisonous by-products of cigarette smoking, is a colourless, odourless gas, which makes up anywhere from 1 to 5 percent of cigarette smoke. It has an extremely strong affinity for haemoglobin, which carries oxygen to all the tissues. Any inhaled carbon monoxide quickly displaces the oxygen in the blood and forms carboxyhaemoglobin. The heart receives less oxygen and has to work harder; it can suffer through damage to the artery walls which then become more vulnerable to the formation of plaque, and the nicotine in cigarettes acts as a stimulant to the adrenal glands to raise blood pressure and heart rate. It all sounds pretty awful, doesn't it? If you're not convinced that there are strong links between smoking and heart disease, have a look at the statistics on page 167.

Most of the large surveys have shown little, if any, increased risk of coronary heart disease in smokers of pipes and cigars; they are mostly light smokers, but those who smoke heavily, or inhale, run an increased risk. Those who change from cigarettes to cigars or pipes may not reduce their risk of disease because they tend to continue to inhale and so maintain levels of carbon monoxide as high as in cigarette smoking. This is most likely to happen in those who smoke small cigars, which yield more tar and nicotine than most brands of cigarettes. The smoke of these cigars may be inhaled just like cigarette smoke.

The question you are probably asking now is will it make any difference if you give up cigarette smoking after a heart attack? Several investigations into this have shown a reduction in the excess risk of heart attack in those who stop smoking compared with those who continue to smoke. It may take ten years or more for ex-smokers to approach the lower risk run by non-smokers. The diagram (p. 168) shows the number of non-fatal relapses after myocardial infarction in a study of 405 patients, comparing continuing smokers with those who had stopped.

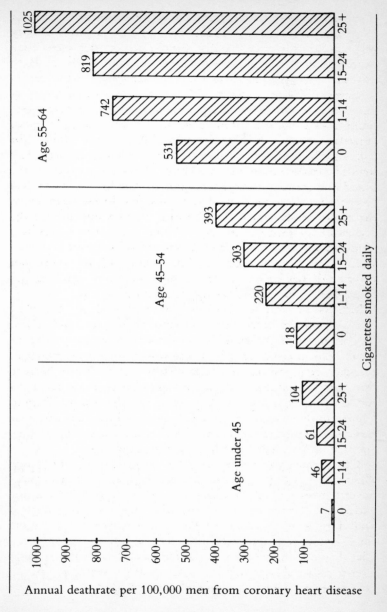

Annual deathrate per 100,000 men from coronary heart disease

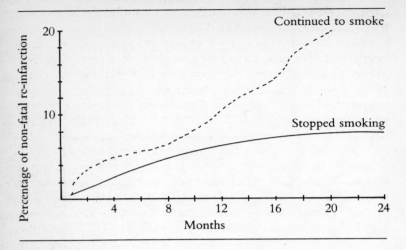

The investigations into smoking and heart disease do not prove that smoking alone actually causes heart disease, but the statistics do show that smoking increases the risk of heart disease by two or three times, compared with people who do not smoke.

c.   *Cholesterol*

Cholesterol is one of several lipids, or fatty acids, found in the blood. In order for the body to transport and use these lipids they must be combined with another molecule to make them soluble in the blood serum (the fluid portion of blood). This molecule is a protein, which combines with the fats to form lipoproteins which vary in size and weight. The heaviest of these molecules is high density lipoprotein (HDL) and is important because it is able to transport fat away from body cells, thus preventing the accumulation of cholesterol and other fats on artery walls. There is evidence that the higher the amount of HDL in the blood, the lower is the risk of atherosclerosis, heart attack and stroke. Women tend to have higher levels of HDL than men and athletes have high HDL, but smokers tend to have low HDL levels. High levels of arousal or stress coupled with fear and anxiety can raise blood cholesterol levels, as do animal fats in the diet.

There are many studies of groups of people, their eating habits and their resulting blood cholesterol levels. Concern about the links between high cholesterol levels and coronary heart disease has a mixed reception among doctors and scientists. There is no clinically measurable level of blood cholesterol above which heart attacks are certain or below which they never occur. But there are facts to support the evidence that the frequency of heart attacks is relatively low in persons who have cholesterol levels below 200 milligrams per decilitre and high in those with cholesterol levels over 300 mg/dl. The highest levels of blood cholesterol are found in North America, central and northern Europe, New Zealand and Australia where the averages range from 220 to 280 mg/dl.

Studies around the world have found that the average cholesterol levels of newborn babies are similar in all population groups – about 65 to 70 mg/dl. But by age 5 to 9 wide disparities among different populations already exist. The affluent Western countries have higher levels of cholesterol than poorer vegetarian countries, and the habits of childhood tend to track on into adulthood.

High levels of blood cholesterol can be lowered by diet. An average reduction in blood cholesterol may be achieved if a new diet provides 30 percent of the calories in fats, no more than 10 percent in saturated fats (animal fats) and if a higher ratio of polyunsaturated fats is adopted. An intake of fibre in the diet and the substitution of vegetable fats or oils for animal protein will reduce cholesterol levels. Another important understanding is the control of weight. Food which is not burned off in exercise can only be stored by the body as fat. Too much fat around the muscles of the heart or in the tissues of the body inevitably puts increased strain on the work of the heart, and lugging more than 10lbs around in overweight takes its toll on the arteries of the limbs and on the circulation generally. Overweight tends also to make us feel depressed and we run the risk of eating even more during these times. There is evidence that an increase in exercise may benefit the body by increasing

HDL which will help to transport cholesterol away from those vital areas.

So how do we know what foods are high in saturated fats and likely to contain more cholesterol than our body can efficiently get rid of? Saturated fat is generally solid at room temperature – for example in bacon, butter, lard, the fat on meat and in hard cheese. There is also about 10 percent fat in milk, eggs and lean beef. Cutting down on these kinds of food products will mean a lower level of blood cholesterol and hopefully a healthier body. Once again, there is not sufficient evidence (as was once thought) to show that high blood cholesterol actually causes coronary heart disease, but its presence does increase the risk. In any event, cutting out a high level of animal fat and dairy produce cannot do any harm, as long as it is replaced with food rich in vitamins and the amount of protein is kept nutritionally sound. Sunflower seed oil instead of lard, rice or grain instead of fried potatoes, fish or vegetables a few times a week instead of meat or cheese . . . this should be sufficient to procude a drop in a raised cholesterol level, and lessen the risk of the excess cholesterol or fat being deposited on artery walls.

d.   Stress

In looking at stress we need to evaluate exactly what we mean by the word stress, what it means to us individually. Many things could be described as stressful but in fact are part of our normal everyday lives. We need to distinguish between healthy, normal stress and tension, without which nothing would get done, and unhealthy stress which, if sustained over long periods causes us distress and forces us to maintain an unnatural stress response for too long a period which leads to fatigue, exhaustion and sometimes breakdown. Levels of stress are examined by looking at our response to the stressor. Flying in an aeroplane, for example, would be highly stressful to some and not to others. We need to look at whether we respond to stress by healthy action which results in a successful outcome, or whether our reaction is fraught with anxiety, fear, struggle against lack of confidence and self-consciousness. It helps to make your own list of personal stress factors in your ordinary everyday life and another list of things which perhaps you avoid because they cause particular stress. Do not forget the stress of worrying, of lack of confidence, fear of the future and of change, that often go unnoticed amongst the host of other matters that occupy our time.

There is evidence, unfortunately only obtained in hindsight, that myocardial infarction is commonly preceded by many months of warning. The important symptoms during this period include abnormal and deepening fatigue which is not removed by sleep; a lethargy and periods of excessive sleeping alternating with sudden bouts of frenzied activity; long hours of working during which little is achieved; minor accidents such as burning a hand over a steaming kettle, breaking a bone in a leg or arm, or dislocating a shoulder. It is as though the body is saying "help, I'm exhausted, give me a rest or a change". Exhaustion is not always an obvious condition which is relieved by a weekend away or a couple of afternoons rest. Real exhaustion goes much deeper than needing a few long sleeps, although sleep is, of course, an important part in the recovery from exhaustion. Dr. Peter Nixon, cardiologist at Charing Cross Hospital writes:

The householder uses a thermostat to help maintain the constancy of the hot water system. The body likewise uses a variety of homeostatic devices to protect the constancy of its internal milieu against the changes which might be caused by our variable responses to the ever-changing circumstances in which we live. Thirst protects us against dehydration, for example, and goose-pimples help to defend us against hypothermia. Fatigue warns us against carrying on until we are exhausted, but the programmes and duties of our lives make us deaf to its voice and our conditioning makes us scorn to listen out for it.

THE HUMAN FUNCTION CURVE (p. 172) is a paradigm illustrating the way we 'go over the hump' into exhaustion and deteriorating function if we allow ourselves to go on being aroused hard and long enough past the level of healthy fatigue. In exhaustion, our trying harder to overcome the deterioration just makes us less efficient because the

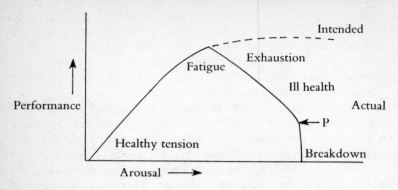

P = The point at which even minimal arousal may precipitate a breakdown.

extra effort increases the arousal, and our performance is already on a downslope. Fighting to close the gap between what we actually can do and what we think is intended of us only widens it. High levels of arousal interfere with the restorative value of sleep and so aggravate the exhaustion.*

So what are the programmes and duties of our lives which force us to press on over the hump into exhaustion? There is no doubt that we live in an extremely complex society with pressures and tensions apparent from the minute we are born, if not well established before birth. Consider the pace at which we expect ourselves to live and our children to grow up, the density and overpopulation of our cities, the competitiveness of education and the struggle to get and maintain jobs, the breaking up of the family unit and of rural communities, the general loss of religion, purpose and meaning which inflict so many lives and forces many to worship money, possessions, speed and indifference. If wonder-drugs have eliminated the diseases feared by our ancestors at the turn of the century, this advance in technology has far outstripped our human ability to cope with change on a fundamental level. Where are the healing arts

* Dr. P.G.F. Nixon, in *The BMA Book of Executive Health*.

today, and the rights and rituals practised as one stage of development passed into another . . . those ritual rights of passage that marked the moving of a boy from adolescence to manhood or a girl into womanhood? The stress of loneliness experienced by those who have been left behind as their family divides and moved away, the difficulty of the old who live longer but have nowhere to go and nothing left to do, the trauma of the youngster who has to look to the Welfare State to offer him structure or mop up his wounds – all this has become so enveloped within the fabric of our lives that we do not notice it anymore; we take it for granted and are puzzled when wise people draw away and talk about stress.

All of us who live in the Western hemisphere live under this kind of stress and add to it individual stresses according to our situation and our personality response. What to one person constitutes stress, to another goes unnoticed, and some people seem to be able to express what they are feeling by bursts of temper and frustration or through the nature of the work they are doing while others bottle it all up inside and live with an intolerable tension.

Some years ago I visited a sausage making factory in Suffolk. Over a hundred girls worked in a large room with machinery going all the time that reminded me of the underground station as the train comes in. They spent twenty minutes on each repetitive activity before changing to another. The smell was appalling, and underfoot was a permanent slippery mess of grease and sausage skins so that you had to be extremely careful how you walked. The noise of the machinery was too loud for them to hear the radio, but it was on full, blaring out hopelessly in all the din. The girls wore surgeon-type gloves to protect their hands and to keep the procedure hygienic. The pace was extremely fast and the conversation was loud and bawdy. There was a rumour that they all trouped off after work and played bingo every night and got drunk as often as possible, and as I left that place I understood exactly why they would want to do both those things . . . to blot out the memory of the day and to drown the horrors of thinking about tomorrow. This work was the only employment for miles, it was well paid and the girls were transported to and from their villages and well looked after.

Similar, and more obvious in many ways, are the stresses experienced by people working in some of the more competitive commercial concerns. The young advertising executive, keen to impress his colleagues and win accounts, often develops an image for himself which is a long, long, way from who he really is underneath and a real gap between personality and behaviour is established. The longer this goes on and the wider the gap, the more difficult it becomes to sustain the image, and this becomes a stress every minute of the day as the struggle to maintain it becomes harder and more desperate. Many people in the commercial world lead Walter Mitty type lives, playing in a game that remains merely that, where their hearts are not in it and their feet do not touch the ground. Huge corporations can produce similar splits in personality, with the individual frantically struggling to be heard, noticed, significant, to 'make it' in order to survive, but against a faceless, depersonalising conglomerate where small individual offerings can so often go unheard.

But we must ask ourselves is this the way we would choose to live . . . and what has this work replaced? And when we have found the answers we have to accept that this is all part of our present day society and that it is stressful – much more stressful for those girls than their ancestors who worked in the fields.

We live in a society that is more informed. We know more about the rest of the world and the way it behaves because we see it on television and read about it in the newspapers. With this new information comes more work for our brains and our understanding. Often in the search for new ideas and enlightenment we forget the bodies that we are dragging along with us; we forget to rest them and energise them by putting them through familiar territory which is nourishment. We forget to be still, and we charge on with adrenalin flowing, stimulation running high, and we become addicted to a fast moving kind of life because this way we feel that we are really living and we are loathe to stop until some event like an illness forces us to be grounded. Many people push themselves way beyond a natural tiredness point and keep themselves going through stimulants like coffee and cigarettes, or they resort to drugs, or they become 'workaholics', addicted to work itself, either through real commitment and love, or from a desire to not have to look too closely at oneself.

Dr. Peter Nixon writes:-

Coronary hypertensive patients are usually preoccupied with the self-defeating struggle to close the gap between what they are actually capable of achieving and what they think they should be achieving. They do not realise that the increments of arousal which increased their performance when they were on the upslope now shift them inexorably downwards, and many cripple themselves unnecessarily or die without learning that the only way back to healthy function is to reduce arousal and remove exhaustion. The interval between the peak and the individual's first cardiovascular breakdown is surprisingly often a period of eighteen months to two years. (See the Human Function Curve on page 172.) High curves enable the individual to withstand a great deal before he becomes exhausted. Conducive to high curves (performance goals) are good mothering; security of support at work and at home; success and the rewards of appreciation and satisfaction; well rooted life in a stable society with knowledge of the cues and responses required for social approval; and the benefits of a training for physical and mental toughness, self discipline and high morale. Low curves predispose to exhaustion, ill-health and breakdown, and coronary mortality is found to be higher when psychological handicaps have created low curves e.g. migration; low grades at school; absent or inadequate parents; lower social status in childhood, growing up in poor areas; lonely isolated uprooted life; and, if a student, being shorter, more tired, older and more disturbed by taxing problems than one's fellows.*

There are other kinds of stress factors which are not always obvious. These are the stresses that come through personal disappointment, disillusionment, loneliness, a sense of worthlessness and pointlessness in life, feelings of isolation, despair, frustration, a feeling of not being able to make it in life, of not being able to cope with relationships, with jobs, with money. These inner feelings may not be communicated to the outside

* *The Practitioner*, Vol. 226, September 1982.

world or shared with other people, but they may take their toll from inside setting up fears and tensions that at times can be unbearable.

The link between stress and coronary heart disease is still debated among doctors and scientists. There is evidence, however, to show the effect of prolonged periods of stress on the blood pressure and on blood chemistry. When we are under stress or anxious our bodies get ready for the 'fight or flight' response. Adrenalin is pumped into the blood so that the muscles are ready for action. If we sustain this pattern for long periods of time we increase the adrenalin, sugar, fat, cholesterol and clotting elements in our blood all of the time, and we increase our susceptibility to heart attack. If, at the same time as having a stressful lifestyle with not enough sleep, we are smoking and drinking to excess in order to keep up, and we are taking little exercise and no relaxation, we are increasing the likelihood of having a heart attack by many times.

My personal view is that we in the twentieth century have yet to fully understand the stress to which we are constantly subjecting ourselves, and I believe that the results of this stress are as yet insidious. There is a feeling of frenzy in the air that will herald the year 2000; there is a feeling of media men gone mad in their search for the most 'over the top' experience. I met a casualty doctor recently who that morning had admitted two young men into intensive care with heart attacks. Both of them were non-smokers, well exercised, relaxed, apparently healthy and happy people. At the time of the attacks one of them, aged 26, staggered out of the horror movie, *The Texas Chain Saw Massacre*, and collapsed in the foyer. The other, aged 32, had had a violent row with his girlfriend and collapsed in Oxford Street. There are other stories, similar to these, and I hear them with alarming frequency. Their study is the subject of another book. But we need to begin asking ourselves . . . what are we doing?

e. *Fatigue and Exhaustion*

or "I"'m so tired I just want to die"

I wonder how many of us take real tiredness seriously: the prolonged, miserable kind of tiredness that isn't relieved by a night's sleep, a weekend break or a holiday. It's the kind of tiredness that won't go away, that forms itself like a fog around us so that we cannot move ... we cannot go forward and we cannot stop, nor can we see what's happening to us. We all get tired ... at best, healthily tired after a day's work or a long stretch of activity, and in a person whose body is working well, this tiredness will be relieved by sleep or time away. And, in the same way, tired spirits will be lifted by a good laugh with friends or a letter from someone we've missed, by happy news and the melancholy felt before will go. But if nothing of this kind relieves your tiredness, in fact, good things such as laughter, beauty, the warmth of companionship, a deep reviving night's sleep, pass you by or do not even exist, then it is likely that you are on the downslope of the Human Function Curve (see preceding section). This means that you have moved from ordinary tiredness into fatigue and the next stage after prolonged fatigue is exhaustion. When we push on through fatigue and exhaustion, trying increasingly harder to make up for our dwindling performance, gathering frustration, a sense of hopelessness, despair and fury at our not accomplishing what we feel we ought, we are pushing against our bodies. This path leads to physical illness and ultimately physical crisis and breakdown.

HOW TO RECOGNISE DANGEROUS FATIGUE

The symptoms of prolonged fatigue likely to lead to exhaustion and breakdown are not easy to recognise because most of us have been taught to look only at actual physical changes in the body such as lumps and spots or pain in a part of the body we can locate. It is also true that most doctors are not trained to look for fatigue, nor do many acknowledge that it is a definite risk factor capable of bringing about change in the physical body and seriously compromising organ function. I talk more about this in the section on stress. There are now an increasing number of studies showing the effects of prolonged exhaustion and the changes produced physiologically. Hopefully, this understanding will become more of an everyday knowledge and help non-medical people to recognise it as a risk factor.

The signs of prolonged fatigue register as follows:

A GRADUAL LESSENING OF PLEASURE.   Food becomes rather tasteless and after we have eaten we still feel unsatisfied; appetite for sex diminishes ... that 'can't be bothered' or putting it off until tomorrow builds up until we can't remember when we last experienced sex or thought about it and it feels a remote event in the past. These things tend not to bother us because all our energy is taken up with keeping going with what we feel we 'have' to do. Enjoyment of simple things – a walk in the country, a warm bath, the smile of a friend – passes us by. Most of these things we don't notice until someone points them out to us and even then this may feel like yet another nag when our life feels already full of nagging. Sometimes it may dawn on us early in morning when we can't sleep that a major event such as the death of a close person, the birth of a child, a major world news item, has actually left us with very little feeling. We have not been really moved. And if we are not naturally cold, this is a horrible shock. We might think "Is this really me?" but not know what to do about it. It is as if we have put our feelings and sensations away somewhere whilst we 'get on' with what we have unconsciously decided must be done at all costs. What happens when we are not in touch with our feelings and sensations is that when they do surface it is always unexpectedly and feelings come out like the eruption of a volcano. We experience unexplained bursts of temper, crying, but, above all, a deep longing for something nice to happen that will make us feel better but which is not met.

INDECISIVENESS.   Not being able to make up our minds within reasonable time and taking much longer than usual about decisions, often on a very mundane and ordinary level, is another sign of prolonged fatigue. For the three years preceding my husband's heart attack, he wore only black ties and the same identical shoes so that he wouldn't have to decide in the mornings. Now he enjoys choosing from a range of colourful ties and takes his time with pleasure. During a period of acute tiredness myself, I wore the same two skirts and sweaters for over a month when I had quite a variety of clothes to choose from but not the inclination. I've seen people so torn between choices and so afraid of not choosing the right one, they spend so much time weighing up each possibility that they do neither but spend the time in a frustrating and anxiety-making funk, feeling worse at not being able to go forward with one choice or the other. Much of the reason for this goes back to the previous section on pleasure. When we are out of touch with our feeling and sensation functions, we don't know what will be nice anymore so we have a hard time deciding what to do.

INCREASE IN SMOKING, DRINKING, EATING AND SPENDING MONEY. Because our selective functioning and being 'at ease' with ourselves has gone into eclipse, we tend to be more obsessive about drink, food, smoking and buying things. They are all attempts to try to feel better, to erase that awful hunger and longing that lies within anyone who suffers from the deprivation which comes from being permanently fatigued with no view of a way out. Unfortunately, the increases we tend to make at this time carry an urgent and obsessive flavour, and in that state we are drawn to instant 'fast' and junk foods full of salt and additives that increase our craving, drive us on to want more and do nothing to diminish our real hunger. Likewise with cigarette smoking, it is not a pleasurable long smoke with a satisfied feel, it is a somewhat manic and desperate lighting up one after another, that starts to happen. We find ourselves in the situation where smoking becomes ritualistic and desperate, as if in a symbolic way we are keeping ourselves together – without it, we would just crumble. And if we have money or not, we find ourselves spending money in that same desperate way. The feeling behind it is: if I buy this dress, house, car, carpet, vase or, nowadays, jogging machine, course of vitamins, special health food for reviving tired muscles, I will feel better, I will be relieved of my exhaustion. A number of the people I have seen over the years have indeed gone the route of buying expensive health cures and health shop remedies or equipment designed to make us fitter, healthier, more relaxed. There are whole new industries which have grown up around this need. But if you are exhausted, a new health cure won't help nor will a change of living place (moving house is high on the Rahe scale of stress), a new dress or perfume. When you are well, these will be great if you can afford them but, for the exhausted person, it's like pouring expensive champagne into a starving baby.

MOOD CHANGES. We experience the extremes of feeling and 'mood'. On the one hand, a heightened, tense, manic kind of excitement where we make all kinds of plans, get fixated on certain ideas, rush around gathering people in to support us, only to forget or move on to another idea the next day; on the other hand, we may experience deep depressive swings which are black and desperate, tinged with cynicism, anger, impotence and self-loathing. Then there are days of nothingness, bland, grey, stuck and monotonous when the whole point of living is lost and a banal 'sameness' covers everything we do. Sometimes we develop paranoia, we feel persecuted by someone or everyone, we feel there are villains everywhere. In extreme cases, exhausted people have been diagnosed as having a paranoid illness and prescribed psychotropic drugs and I have seen patients come into hospital carrying just this label who, when slept and rested, are receptive to the ideas of rehabilitation and all signs of paranoia are gone. What is probably true is that the tendencies or characteristics that we all have uniquely, become exacerbated by exhaustion as they do by alcohol. Someone who behaves a little suspiciously or in a paranoid way may be pushed into more severe displays of this tendency under the pressure of fatigue.

FEELING TRAPPED. We can get into several different traps – emotional, work, housing, friendship – and the physical trap of overwork and fatigue. When we realise we are trapped, we may fight to get out and to resolve our predicament. If this fails, we can't get out, we can't go forward or go back to where we started, we feel frightened, furious, despairing, impotent and helpless. People react in different ways according to their personalities and upbringing. Some people accept their situation with a saintly resignation: "There's nothing we can do." But the despair and anger seethe away inside, not always consciously. Others produce resentment, anger which becomes disabling and turns inward against themselves and a despairing bitterness which makes others shun them and send sympathies elsewhere. Some people assume a martyrish role, submerging themselves and their needs in an increasingly tyrannical fashion, unaware of the ways they are using their energy, but often projecting their anger and helplessness onto others, producing a great deal of guilty feelings. But overall, feeling trapped makes us try to work harder to get out and, if we are blinded by fatigue and some of the feelings described above, we can fight against ourselves trying to fly away and crash, like Icarus, broken winged, exhausted and defeated. We may well be in a different trapped situation – an unhappy marriage, a difficult job, stuck with an unwanted invalid – but fighting against our situation only exacerbates our fatigue.

DEPRESSION. Clinical depression and fatigue have very similar symptoms and are often impossible to separate because they are so often intertwined. My work is to look at both issues and try to determine what are the triggering factors that lead people into a depressed and exhausted state. Some people get depressed because of their predicament which may be outlined by any of the states described above. Some people may be exhausted by their depression, by a constant anxiety state, a lack of assertiveness, a vulnerable personality, weak ego structure, poor background, lack of confidence, lack of bonding with another person. It is the part of them which is struggling to be free of their exhaustive and depressed trap which needs to be held and helped to channel itself creatively, so that the results are more encouraging, more positive. When people know that being exhausted exacerbates their depressed feelings, they feel less trapped by the depression itself and, in particular, any psychiatric label they may have been given. Understanding about lifestyle and habits, breaking down just where areas of difficulty lie, where the lack of assertiveness presents itself, looking at just how the person manages his or her life and difficulties, can give an exhausted and depressed person something more to go on than their looking only at the four walls of their trap or their psychiatric label. Many people in this state tend to look at huge issues, they look at the whole week ahead and fear getting through it, rather than what they need to do in the next hour which is much more manageable. The important issue to focus on is that it is not the *whole* of us which gets stuck, exhausted, depressed, psychotic, it is a PART of us that has for some reason been driven that way. Seeing this as a part allows us to examine that part and to recognise it when we see it taking over. Knowing this also means we have it, not it having us!

SITUATIONS LIKELY TO LEAD TO FATIGUE AND EXHAUSTION

DIFFICULT RELATIONSHIPS. We all know about "Who's afraid of Virginia Woolf" type relationships, couples who are locked together in an invisible web of love and hate, with more expression of the hate and loathing than the love. Sometimes hate is a more powerful bond than love and people stay together for years for what would seem the flimsiest of reasons. "I wouldn't let him get away with divorce after the way he's been," one woman said to me of her husband's infidelities. "We've got to stay together because of the children" is a very frequent assumption, even when children have said they would prefer the couple to separate because of the awful situation at home. Evidence from studies of divorced families suggests that, in some very destructive situations, children are happier and develop better when their parents have separated and are leading more normal and more relaxed lives.

Many people find themselves left looking after a relative or difficult old parent and wonder how it all happened, they feel caught out of duty and often love but do not feel free to talk about their difficulties or get too tired to seek or ask for help. Some people blame themselves for getting into relationships that no longer work and leaving is not an option they feel they have because of religious or moral views, fears of the partner they would be leaving, loss of social position, money, prestige, friends, security and often one thing – a favourite pet, the garden shed, an aged relative – keep people in relationships that have become destructive.

Our emotional reactions to those we are intimately involved with, even if destructively, have a powerful effect upon our body and, in particular, our hearts. You only have to look at a patient's blood pressure chart at visiting time. Some charts are raised by twenty points due to the stress of the visit and the pressure the patient is put under. Some people seem to be addicted to each other; they haven't a good word to say about the other person but they can't leave them alone. It becomes as if they need this daily dose of adrenalin, fury, blood boiling, bile spitting and venom and both people are caught in it. These types of relationships come to a head when one person becomes ill. Their illness may become a weapon and is used as such; the other partner may not be able to stop themselves acting as before, only now with more guilt and more internalised anger. Their resentment at the other person getting ill and getting attention may push them further apart at the same time as the new situation, the current ill health, forces them together. This can become a locked situation where counselling can help. It is vital to facilitate a greater objectivity into a painful and 'fixed' situation. There may be no answer to many life problems and no clear way out but outside resources can often be found to offer support and understanding, even if there is no possibility for change.

POOR SLEEPING HABITS.   Poor sleeping habits may come about because of worry. And there may be times when our sleep is interrupted. After a baby is born, for example, or during illness or looking after a sick relative or child who needs our attentions in the night. Current worries or fears may keep us awake at night as well as practical realities. When our sleep is broken several times during the night, for whatever reason, we don't get our proper, deep sleep and, although we may be able to carry on in this way for some time, we are running ourselves on reserve tanks of energy which soon get used up. It is true also that poor sleep itself worries us, that we begin to fear going to sleep in case we don't sleep properly and so it is the fear of not sleeping itself which may contribute to keeping us awake. If you have a period of worry or have to take charge of someone who is ill and needs you in the night, try to plan it all as you would an expedition. Know that you are carrying this added burden and accept it willingly as such. Know that in your current situation you are going to feel tired and must take it into account. Know this when you are offered invitations or plan travelling or outings, accept visitors, take on an extra little job. Make it an 'event', something tangible, rather than running along trying not to notice it or as if it didn't matter. It does matter, and not sleeping takes away the stores of energy we need for a day. Take any chance you can of resting and sleeping at different times. On the bus, sitting waiting, even in queues you can close your eyes for a minute or two. It's as if you are saying to your body: here you are, here's a chance for some refuelling. Ask for help from people, someone to take turns to help look after the person who may be ill, someone to share your worry with. It always helps to talk over a problem with someone else or to write it all down so that you can get some focus onto it, you get things into proportion. It may be that you need medical help from a doctor when poor sleeping becomes a problem. It is worth taking medication even if you basically don't like to, perhaps for a week to get your body properly rested and slept so that you may get out of a bad sleeping cycle. You may also be helped by taking herbal teas.

LACK OF SELF-ESTEEM.   Lack of self-esteem is what may lie behind our tiredness and exhaustion. As well as carrying out our daily tasks, we carry the extra load of fear and worry that we might make a mistake, something that goes wrong will be our fault, we will lose our job if we put but a foot wrong; we may have difficulty sustaining relationships, we may never be assertive or like to ask for anything for ourselves because we feel we are not worth it and that no-one will care for us anyway. Lack of self-esteem then undercurrents everything that we do, can actually make life very much more difficult for us, give us a feeling that we are walking uphill all the time. If you feel you suffer from lack of self-esteem, you may be helped by Chapter 6 of this book, by finding out for yourself just where your poor self-esteem is located, where it comes from and what you might do about improving the situation.

have shown that a person with 'A Type' Behaviour is prone to heart disease.

I speculate that one of the reasons the 'A Type' man hurries and runs *through* life to the exclusion of living *in* life is that he is in essence running away from what he sees as his inferior self. The more that 'life' tries to slow him down or challenge him to change, the more he gets 'stuck' in to the 'hurry sickness', and the more off-balance he becomes in terms of the conscious and unconscious forces of the psyche. It is possible that the twentieth century person who conscientiously pursues achieve-ment goals set for him by society and his environment to the detriment of his own inner and private world, is doing so because the power of both extremes is too great for him to balance the two. Many of the people I spoke to in cardiac wards spoke of their dream and fantasy life with great fear and wonder. Many of them knew on one level what might be revealed to them were they to respond to the unconscious, and they feared that it might pull them out of control, that they might never 'get back' to take care of the projects they had set themselves. With each unconscious – i.e. dream or idea – revelation, they threw themselves with even more frenzy into the things they knew, doing them more quickly and less well, building up frustration and anxiety and eventually despair. One man said to me: "I kept having these dreams, about missing a train. It wasn't an ordinary train but a very beautiful one, lit up with fairy lights and decked with wonderful flowers. However fast I ran I could never catch up with it. Sometimes I would think about that train during the day at work. I got frightened when I realised the tricks my mind was playing. My daydream-ing got me into several accidents. I thought I was losing my marbles."

Many patients identified themselves with their jobs, their possessions, their wives and children, their achievements out in the world. Lying flat on their backs in a hospital bed and being nursed they were stripped of everything they knew and became very vulnerable and tearful. Could this regression to an infant-like stage be a bid for things to begin again, to be born again, with a new identity? The insecurity of being in this state is felt most acutely by the man or woman who has made material success and achievement their gods, for they have no resources with which to deal with the time they now have on their hands, and with the emotion that fills their waking moments. Very often this 'type' of person – most commonly recognised as the 'type' most likely to suffer heart attack in the forties: the overweight, overworked, business executive desperately climbing his ladder but never being satisfied with the height he has reached – has been unable to ask for any kind of help throughout life. Because he has placed more value on the creation of external merits and on the 'number game' (the accumulation of numbers of things done, money made, operations performed, etc.), he has not been in touch with the admiration or respect of his colleagues or friends, or with any of the feeling qualities that surround what he does. These things are unknown ground to him; he has little use for them, in others or in himself. But after a heart attack it is these feeling qualities that are being asked to come to the surface. The very real question of "who am I?" is asked over and over again. If you are ill and helpless what use are your fleet of motor cars or millions of dollars in the bank?

If a man's hostility and aggression are raised by his competitive reaction to the demands of his environment he spends his time being 'big and brave', raising and tightening his chest against the world. What he fears most are his feelings and his 'inner' life, and he deals with this anxiety in a cloud of cigarette smoke or the speed of his motor car. He is fighting against his own body, he may even try and run past death itself. Many patients have described to me their feelings of being 'cut off' from sensation, 'not being able to feel anything' prior to their heart attacks. Some said that they often felt so tense that they thought they would burst. At the time they could not understand what it meant and they got on with the work they knew so well even more furiously. But in the atmosphere of care and love of a therapeutic hospital, or better still, at home, these things can be shared and pondered over, and at this time there is an overwhelming response by the heart attack victim to the old fashioned virtues of listening, kindness and gentleness.

h.   Symptom as Symbol

When body and mind lose their connecting links, we act unconsciously as the effect of this disconnection continues internally. This happens when an event in life is too great to be assimilated by the mind, and so the memory and feeling of the event is carried by the body unconsciously. We all know of people who express one thing with their words and a quite different thing with their bodily expression.

We know that there is a mysterious 'leap' from mind to body which underlies hysterical conversion and the various inhibitions of bodily functioning. The form of our psychic productions is determined by the way in which the psyche is structured, and they have meaning in relation to our wish to live, and to go on with our lives as best we can with what we are given. In an attempt to maintain psychic equilibrium every human being is capable of producing neurosis, perversion, dream and fantasy and creative works of art. The way in which we work with the creative potential of these psychic manifestations determines the psyche's safety and balance. When psychic messages are ignored for a long period and we fail to maintain some kind of equilibrium to deal with psychic pain, the psychosomatic process may take over and somatic, biological illness may form. It is the body which is pulling the psyche and soma together as a whole, or attempting to.

If we look only at the external symptoms of heart disease and evaluate its cause according to the physiology of the body, the only advice we would have to offer a heart patient would be to stop smoking, lose weight or change his eating habits and take more exercise. These activities have proved that they can contribute to a healthier life. Looking at the symptom as a symbol for some inner psychic need, we could ask "what does your heart mean to you?", or "what does the word heart mean for you?" or "when you think of the pain in your heart, what does it remind you of?". We could then get a picture of what part the disease was playing in the life of the individual, what it was saying to him about his life, and it would give us clues as to how to help this patient in a complete, holistic, sense. Using the body as the centre of meaning we may locate hidden or repressed feelings which have communicated themselves to consciousness through physical pain. The 'body memory' can then communicate what is the source of pain and a way to heal this can be found through therapy. Behaviour patterns that have 'blocked off' or disguised some precious vulnerability during a period in the past, may be questioned and reformed. Old defences, which were valid at a needful time but which are still being used, may be eased away. An appreciation of the individual need for taking responsibility for both psychic and physical health may begin to develop. Change may be accepted as an imperative for healing and growth. An acceptance of and an understanding of the balance of the psyche and soma will greatly aid recovery after illness, whether or not accompanied by medication.

It is my understanding that every symptom tells a story and that the underlying myth of the premature heart attack is one of death and rebirth; a bid to end a psychological death and begin again. But the level of despair and loneliness that accompanies the journey through this experience means that there is a high risk of actual physical death. We need to know more about the silent messages of the body, our own and other people's. We need to study body language and recognise the body's memory. We need to have a true reverence for the impact of the mind upon the body before the body takes over and does its own 'thinking'.

James Lynch writes:

If living patterns and human companionship do influence the incidence of cardiovascular disease, then it would appear that medicine has been misdirecting its preventative skills. A few heart transplants receiving world-wide attention have led to widespread euphoria – in just a few more years, perhaps, everyone will be able to receive new hearts, just as we replace worn-out tyres on cars. It should be pointed out, however, that no-one has yet suggested opening a 'spare parts' department store for worn-out or defective human emotions. The repair of the 'broken heart' from the loss of a loved one may present far more of a therapeutic challenge than the technical skills needed for a heart transplant operation.*

i. *Obesity and Heredity*

OBESITY

Obesity means being heavier than the average for one's height, age and sex, based on the standardised weight tables produced largely for insurance companies' guidelines. Surveys based on insurance company recordings indicate that the death rate from all causes, including cardiovascular ones, rises as relative weight goes from low to above average and the increase is substantial in people whose weight is 30% above average. Most of the relationship between obesity and coronary heart disease is with angina rather than heart attack or coronary death. Other problems associated with obesity are high blood pressure, diabetes and high blood uric acid which tend to disappear after weight reduction.

HEREDITY

There are hereditary facts which shows a tendency to coronary artery disease, namely a high lipid disorder known as familial hypercholestercemia. This is characterised by very high levels of cholesterol in the blood. Fortunately this tendency is rare. In some families where several members have died of heart attacks or strokes at a relatively early age, it is obviously important to pay attention to preventative measures and avoid the known risk areas. A tendency to hypertension and diabetes would seem to be inherited and both these factors earn a cardiovascular risk. It seems that habits such as smoking, over-eating, little exercise and a tendency to 'A type' personality pursuits may also be inherited but by learned behaviour rather than genetic definition.

* *The Broken Heart*; Lynch, J.L., Harper & Row (1977).

Chapter 8

Families and Couples

a. *What Do We Tell the Children?*

DURING MY WORK AS a therapist, I have met many people with childhood memories of father, mother, grandfather, grandmother, uncles and aunts who 'had a bad heart'. This was synonymous with: 'be careful', 'talk in whispers', 'never raise your voice in their presence or do anything disagreeable, like shout or sing, make whooping noises, or dance on the table'. Even handstands in the garden were forbidden in one case. At the severe end of this scale, children can grow up picking up the message ... don't be yourself ... don't express yourself ... and if you do ... someone will die. You can see that these are extremely powerful messages to ingest along with Marmite and Ribena. Later on in life, they can lead to disturbances such as phobic avoidance of any kind of creative activity; holding the breath, which can lead to hyperventilation and to chest pain and coronary spasm, thus repeating the pattern of heart disturbance through the generation. It can lead to phobia about death, fears of all kinds, particularly ill-health, and tremendous sense of guilt if anything goes wrong with health in the family.

TAKING 'MAGICAL' GUILT means that you take on board the responsibility of whatever ills happen in the family – including mother or father's bad heart. When something bad happens, you feel as if it is your fault, and you creep away feeling bad inside or bad about whatever it was you said or did. Taking on 'magical' guilt in this way can lead us to suspend our lives later on, feeling that we have no 'rights' to assert ourselves or do our own thing, we are afraid of our own power, or our own ambitions, wants, creativity, our own wishes ... they have become confused with "If you carry on in this way ... someone will get ill or, worse, die because of it."

You can see that after a heart attack in the family, it is extremely important to be clear with children about what is happening. Explain to them what the patient can do or not do. Explain to them how they can help with the situation, rather than instructing them in what not to do. Practical things: "you be grandpa's legs for him for a bit" ... "will you help us by bringing in the coal/carrying the shopping/making the tea/answering the telephone," are far preferable than shushing and silencing. Children pick up fear very quickly even if no words are spoken. When you get home from hospital explain to the children what needs to happen ... even the littlest needs to know ... the two-and-a-half-year-old as well ... how the convalescent period is to be structured ... that from two till four in the afternoon is quiet time, when father or mother are sleeping and need quiet ... phones are taken off the hook, no TVs or radios are allowed and so on. The other times should be as normal as possible in terms of everyday life. Inevitably, as we've been discussing in this book, moods change and swing about a bit after a heart attack and sometimes children get on the end of such changes, perhaps becoming the target for irritability, depressed thinking, anger and rage. Something small that a child does can trigger off underlying tension. Know this and allow for it, explaining to a child that it is not all his fault but that dad, mum or whoever is having a hard time. It is important too that children can speak freely to a parent who has been ill in this way, that they do not feel they have to swallow their feelings towards the parent just because the person 'has a bad heart'. We are all human and we need to remember this, and a person with a bad heart can make someone just as angry as someone who has a healthy one, and it's appropriate to be angry sometimes, and good for the person to realise they are not 'special' just because of their illness.

CHILDREN ARE GOOD AT STORIES AND MYTH-MAKING.   It is only too easy for children to weave some fantastic fabrication around what is happening in the family if it is not demystified. One little boy was reported saying to his younger sister aged four: "If you play your mouth organ near grandma, her heart will jump right out of her body and get stuck up on that tree and the birds will peck it for their dinner." The little girl threw her mouth organ in the dustbin. One girl had had to walk around the house talking only in whispers for all of her childhood because raised voices might start grandma off on another 'turn'. Later on in life she could rarely make herself heard by anyone, and compensated by developing a shouting voice, forced out from her upper chest. This made her breathing difficult and she started hyperventilating, leading on to chest problems of her own.

CHILDREN NEED TO BE TOLD EVERYTHING in a language they can understand, and they need to be watched very carefully after a heart attack in the family, in case they are building up problems inside themselves that will become serious later on.

b. Couples

It sometimes happens that when one person in a couple gets a heart complaint, the physical problem brings to the surface a great deal of bitterness and resentment from both the patient and his partner. If the relationship has been struggling before, now is the time when these struggles feel unbearable. The person with the suffering heart may blame the other person for putting too much pressure on them, not giving them enough space for themselves, they may feel unloved, uncherished, unappreciated, hurt by the other, furious with the other, resentment toward the other, and yet none of these feelings may have been openly acknowledged before. They may have been bottled up for years and, coupled with frustration and bitterness of this, may actually have been threatening homeostasis with their accompanying blood chemistry changes. In the other camp, the partner may be seething with fury that he or she has never been properly heard by the other, that her views, feelings, anger, rage and frustration have disappeared into a controlling refusal to be recognised. In the chapter on anger, we talked about the 'holier than thou' attitude which can grow from unexpressed anger. This can be infuriating to someone who is trying to communicate what they feel and gets pushed away as irrelevant all the time.

Another situation is one in which there is a cold, unyielding quality within the partnership. Where the 'stiff upper lip' approach is prevalent, where life is valued by doing rather than being, by external successes and appearances rather than the quality of life. One partner may have suppressed his or her desire for a more feeling relationship in order to keep up appearances (many marriages, which were made before 1939 or in the early days after the war, do carry this flavour with them ... 'one does what one has to do'), but the other does not see why anything should be any different. As the years go by, the gulf caused by this difference gets wider and different problems emerge. Both partners are, in fact, denying the value of expressing feeling and human need in relationship. Becoming ill in the heart – the symbolic seat of the feeling function – may be one way of drawing attention to the needs of the heart – to be held, to be warm, to be loved and accepted, wanted and cherished. The heart may be crying out in despair for the coldness, aloofness and hurt in the unforgiving atmosphere of a marriage built on convenient arrangement rather than love.

Some people seem destructively bound up with each other, and more so as time goes on. If a message of the heart (see Chapter 2 on "Why? And what does it mean?") does not get listened to or appreciated as something shared within the relationship, the situation intensifies and people get more stuck, more destructive, more furious with each other, less able to give anything at all. As the sickness in the heart remains unresolved, a new pattern of resentment can begin to get built up ... resentment by the other for all the time and attention the 'patient' receives ... the sympathy from others, which can often seem to push the partner more into isolation, making their feelings further away and less likely to be voiced. Whereas before, the couple may have been searching for something to bring them closer together in understanding, now, they have an illness within them that invariably throws them together but in a negative way. If both members of the partnership are prepared to share this problem, a great deal can be done through good counselling to help their plight. Sadly, so often the patient tries to grab all the sympathy from outside to justify his hurt from his partner, or the partner feels trapped in a web of fear and guilt, pushing her fury further down and away. Or, the patient may be the one who realises what is happening but be unable to communicate to the other person, or the person is not able to listen or to change.

We weave complex tangles as adults in our human relationships. Couples share the same adrenalin levels, the same arousal levels and often the same coping strategies. Heart patients are notoriously tough in terms of endurance and stoicism. If this energy could be channelled into creating a better environment for relationship, by realising that if the individual problem is getting stuck in a trap door or on the treadwheel, getting exhausted by soldiering on, then much of the rhythm of the marriage or partnership will have taken on this flavour. An individual can be stopped, helped to take stock and see what resources are available for help. Couples can do just the same. Actually stop. Stop the habitual remark, the habitual coping strategy when the going gets tough and defences are raised through behaviours which are really saying "don't hurt me" ... If you recognise that you are in a trap like this in your relationship and your heart is doing the talking for you, take yourself and your partner to the most experienced counsellor or therapist in couples work that you can find, and start to unravel exactly what is happening. (Useful reading – *Families – How to survive them* by Robin Shynner & John Cleese.)

c.   How Families Cope

The family network takes on much of the burden of change associated with learning to recover properly after a heart attack. Whether the family is just one couple with the cat, whoever is at home after the heart attack patient returns from hospital or convalescence is involved in recovery, and this affects everyone from babies and animal pets to grandmothers, aunts and cousins. Many of the doctors I spoke to said they felt they didn't do enough to help the families. So often there wasn't time to talk or explain, and apart from the follow-up appointment after returning home many people didn't see their doctor at all. Some GPs do indeed call regularly on patients after a hospital admission and questions can be answered then. Some district nurses, community nurses and social workers get involved visiting families after serious illness and these visits are a valuable resource for families who feel cut off from information and support. In their studies with patients and their wives after myocardial infarction Dr. Stephen Jordan and Mrs Carol Trelawny-Ross report the following:

Thirty-two men and their wives discussed their experiences of admission to hospital and subsequent rehabilitation following a threatened or confirmed myocardial infarction. Over all, the level of information and understanding about their condition was poor. Patients would have liked to have had more specific advice about rehabilitation and to have been told more about their condition. Thirteen discharging doctors indicated on a short questionnaire what advice they had given to their patients. This exercise confirmed the suspicion that while patients' memory might have been poor, they had not been given extensive information before they left hospital. In particular, although all of the men were married and under sixty-five years of age, only 38% of the doctors said that they had discussed sexual activity and of the whole sample (32 men) only 25% of the men recalled having been advised on this subject. Patients and their wives felt that they would have worried less if they had been better informed. Persistent symptoms were related more to worry and depression than to the extent of myocardial damage.*

In any crisis information is vital. Families need to have detailed information about what is happening whilst their family member is in hospital and their need to be around when information is given about rehabilitation afterwards. This helps the situation to be shared, and during shock we tend not to remember details very well. If we are frightened by something we tend to block it out in order to cope. Until we can take things on board families are an important resource in assisting patients during their everyday

---

* Do we tell our coronary patients enough? Carol Trelawny-Ross, M.Sc, Stephen Jordan, FRCP. From the Department of Mental Health, University of Bristol and the Cardiac Department of the Bristol Royal Infirmary, 1986.

activities. As we've said before in this book – write down the problems or questions as they occur and before a visit from a professional decide what you want to ask. Make a list of priorities as there are likely to be many small queries during the early days. Try and gather everyone in the family to make suggestions – everyone has a valid contribution to make and the more people involved in help, the stronger the support system and the more freedom each individual member has to go about his or her own life. If you take it in turns to help out, the load is spread and shared. One family I knew worked out a rota system for someone to be in the house all the time during the first two weeks after the grandmother had had a serious infarction. The times were deliberately kept short, so that no one had to do a long period of time in, and because it was shared democratically, there was no resentment. Some people find information about recovery hard to get, from hospitals or GPs. It helps to be persistent and you do have the right to ask.

Chapter 9

Counselling the Exhausted at Heart

IN MY WORKSHOPS I talk about the 'worker' heart – the pump responsible for keeping blood circulating around the body; and the 'feeling' heart – the symbolic partner through whose centre feelings flow in and out in a similar circulatory way. We all, at one time, have touched our hearts when we expressed strong feelings of love, pain, joy, loss, and we use the word heart in our language – heartfelt, heartsick, lionheart, faintheart, "don't wear your heart on your sleeve". We all know that our hearts beat faster when we are close to those we love, or when we feel hurt or offended by them. We feel our heart heavy with the loss of a loved one; it turns over in ecstasy and pleasure; it soars when we are happy, and most of us know what it's like to have our heart pressed as if by some crushing weight at times of pain and difficulty. And our use of language to describe a feeling has now been scientifically correlated. When the heart beats faster during strong emotion, adrenalin is produced from the adrenal glands and catecholemine changes are found in the blood. Some of these chemical changes are advantageous, they set us in motion, and the flight-or-fight response has been our main survival mechanism from our earliest of days. However, long-term, continual excitation of these hormonal responses to emotion, particularly negative emotion such as despair, defeat, isolation, helplessness, a sense of hopelessness, can actually over-ride the natural balance-restoring properties in the body and produce permanent chemical change in the tissues. This is a quantifiable, scientific proven link between the body and mind in relation to the heart.

Counselling can begin at any time an individual realises they have a problem carrying, coping or expressing what is going on in their emotional life, and that this is affecting their relationship to people and their health.

Some people who have had a heart attack can take in information about what has happened to them, look at what attitudes or behaviour contributed to bringing on the attack and, with basic help and training in breathing techniques, relaxation techniques, understanding the proper use of effort, and reprioritising their lifestyle, can make good changes necessary for healthy recovery. In fact some people find recovery from a heart attack a positive challenge to get more out of their lives and start doing the things they most enjoy in a new, heartfelt way. People have said to me: "I was lucky ... I've had a warning, now I am on borrowed time ... it's a bonus, a gift, and I must use it well, not waste time getting cross about things that don't matter, arguing with people out of pride or out-of-date principles, worrying about things I can't do anything about." And many people do make these adjustments to enjoy their lives and their families.

But for some people the negative input persists. The inner voice that nags 'you haven't done enough ... you haven't got it right ... you watch out or X will overtake you ... you must have X amount of money in the bank or you won't be safe'. All these kind of inner voices or messages serve to force an individual on, often irrationally and unrealistically, against what they might choose to do were they free of such voices. And less specific, feelings of inadequacy, low self-esteem, fears of all kinds, of being left behind, excluded, of being lonely, abandoned, are behind the drive for people to keep going on their particular treadwheel. Counselling can help to isolate the messages that drive people on inappropriately, to find out where they come from, who they belong to, and help an individual to separate out which voice is responsible for his behaviour patterns and give him a choice whether or not to listen. New voices can be born in this situation. Voices of encouragement, permission and hope can awaken a sense of the original seed within the person, which has been eclipsed by more strident, driving, negative forces built in at an early age. Ongoing counselling can help to strengthen the true voice of the individual so that he can stand up to the critical negative voices inside and begin to live his own life more fully, more appropriately. Sometimes this process takes time and one of the problems that both counsellor and client come up against is the urgent nature of the driving negative force inside the person, which sometimes urges them to give up the 'self indulgence' of looking at themselves. More and more people are beginning to recognise that attitude and behaviour are linked with health and are beginning to take a look at what is available to help themselves. This is good, but there is no quick solution. Firmly entrenched attitudes which become 'known' to be destructive don't go away after one session of therapy or by 'knowing' what it's all about. There is no quick headache cure for people with a long history of being dominated by negative input about themselves and this is sometimes a problem to people whose whole life is one big rush. It is not enough to say to someone "If you carry on like this, you will die prematurely." They won't believe you. Skilled counselling needs to get behind these hurrying defences and harness the positive, creative energies, and not antagonise the defences into further entrenchment by full frontal challenge. Enlightenment can be quick ... heart patients tend to be an intense, intelligent, diligent and tough lot, they really work, and they realise what is going on inside them quickly. The real work begins after enlightenment, in terms of trying new ways, or not giving in destructively to the well-worn driving forces in the personality. It hurts sometimes to get off the track and it can be frightening. All those demons people were running away from in the first place have to be faced: "If I am not seen to be successful/ to always get it right/be perfect/always top, no one will notice/ love/like/see me ever again." These reasons, however irrational when first realised, are very powerful indeed. The fears have to be faced, the ghosts named and faced, if they are to disappear and leave room for true self to emerge. Compulsive behaviours are built as defence mechanisms for very important reasons. Early in life we need to defend ourselves from emotions we can't handle at the time. A child who has no place to put his frightened and lonely feelings because no one listens, will cover them up by perhaps rushing around making a lot of noise, or pleasing people by doing what they want in order to get their approval and hopefully their love. Later on, in his thirties or forties, he may be doing the same thing automatically, as if there was still no one to listen. But things outside may well have changed, and what has changed is that he is no longer four years old but may have more resources to get or ask for help. His habitual defence then is actually redundant but he doesn't realise it, and he needs to get used to the idea and try out what it feels like for his ground rules to be different.

Counselling can have different phases:

1   Education of the links between body and mind in relation to the heart. Encouragement of self-monitoring of pulse and blood pressure. Teaching breathing and relaxation techniques.

2   Looking at and mapping our lifestyle, roles played, energy needed.

3   Recognition of inner voices. What is it that drives the person on in different areas?

4   Presumption of absolutes in life, i.e. if I am not seen to be in control, perfect all the time, I will be nothing, rubbished by other people; or, if I am not always nice, smiling and do what people want, no one will love me, like me, or accept me, or even see me.

5   Helping people to look at body language. Times when they raise shoulders, tighten buttocks and back, clench fists etc. Finding out what this means ... cigarette smoking and compulsive eating come into this area also. Look at what it means.

6   Current lifestyles and habits in relation to the sense of 'real' self as this begins to emerge. Does the life, job, qualities etc., suit the needs of the individual, or are people living out past parental expectations?

7   Assessment of coping skills. For some people overwork or compulsive behaviours are a way of coping with shock or change, and this includes coping with having a heart attack. With a greater sense of inside strength, other tactics of dealing with external stresses can be tried rather than the automatic taking off at full steam. Many people need to be

helped to assess their coping skills by looking at different events in their lives, times to conflict, and help in appraising what helped them through, what parts of themselves they perhaps were using without realising or valuing. This gives choice in terms of coping. Many people need help to assess their external resources, particularly if they are of the type that don't like to ask for help from others. They may find there are many more people or skills available and all they have to do is overcome their fear of the consequences of asking. Sometimes mapping out support and resource systems is useful, making lists of people available or basic information of who or what is around in different areas to offer help.

Basic self-assertion techniques can be learnt when people feel they 'are allowed' to have a life of their own free from negative treadmill constraints. They can also claim their right to pleasure, relaxation, fun, holidays and just 'being' time, which they cannot claim without guilt and more compulsive behaviour when they are under the spell of negativity.

When the person is receptive to ideas about caring for himself and has begun to feel that it is actually worth it, understanding about rest and sleep, diet and exercise, meditation and relaxation are useful tools to help him maintain homeostasis and to enhance his new found feelings of well-being. At some point, I always ask a person "Why do you think you had a heart attack?" Inside they always know. Use of imagery, active imagination, guided imagery and drawing can help to anchor the imaginative products of people's souls and connect them with something of meaning inside themselves, something that is truly of them, originally, that they can ponder on and go back to at times of vulnerability or need. So often the psyche throws up a dream or an image that, when amplified, can help people to understand their next step, or which clears an understanding of a part of themselves previously under-rated or unexplored.

There is a possibility that our epidemic of heart problems has something to do with the Western collective polarisation of thinking and feeling. We live in a time when there is a split between head and heart. We overvalue the rational, logical binary thought processes which dominate government, education and medicine and the heart centred values of love and containment, imagination, pondering, stillness, reflection tend to be under-valued and left out. Somewhere man's soul is starving. And where can these rejected and devalued feelings go but into the body of the heart itself. Alfred Zeigler writes:

Somatisation is inconceivable unless it is preceded by a 'going astray' of our particular talents. Nature seems to tolerate only a limited measure of onesidedness. When the limits are exceeded, or if too much energy is devoted to onesidedness, nature counterbalances the tendency through our bodies, as seeking a more effective or impressive means of demanding recognition for her chimerical plans.*

* Alfred Zeigler: *Archetypal Medicine*.

Conclusion

You will cull from this book what is important, necessary to you and your life *now*. And it will be personal and relevant to you. My hope is that a phrase or sentence may start you off on an inner personal journey which results in your having something in your life beyond that which your body has produced, a greater sense of yourself, of meaning, of your place in the world. A heart attack is a product of the world we live in, a symptom of the stress and distress of the society we have created. We can't change society overnight, but we can change and develop our own personal input; individually, one by one, so that ultimately a major shift is experienced. Our concern in this book has been with the individual, the person who has had a heart attack and each person around them, whose life has also been changed by the experience.

We must learn to live now. We must learn to catch ourselves when we are nearing the repetition of the treadmill existence and understand the dangers this has for us if we persist in the "when I've . . . I'll start living". That day never comes; there is always another hill to climb, another river to cross, another bridge to build. And this is well and good, it is the stuff of our life if we embrace it consciously with a spirit of adventure. There is an urgency which comes with the struggle to find identity, meaning, purposefulness, love, acceptance. These things are not ever found outside; they come from within, when there is a meeting with inner realisation, and outer struggles are put within this context. The sense of time – urgency, of desperately looking for recognition and the 'numbers game' of the 'A type' personality, put us on a rocky path to an unhappy, premature death.

The only resource we have is the person we see in the mirror every morning. This is the resource we need to value and know and understand as intimately as we can. Doctors may sew up our wounds, nurses tend us as lovingly as an infant and their specialised knowledge offer us a safe sanctuary during illness, but this is only a beginning. It is never too late to look in the mirror afresh.

Notes

p. 186. 'Physiological responses to psychological challenge under hypnosis in patients considered to have hyperventilation syndrome: complications for diagnosis and therapy.' Leisa J. Freeman, MB; MRCP Research Fellow Ashley Conway, BSc., Hypnotherapist, Peter G.F. Nixon, FRCP, Consultant Cardiologist Cardiac Department, Charing Cross Hospital.

Reading

HEART

'A Type' Behaviour and your Heart, Meyer Friedman, M.D. & Ray Rosenman, M.D.

Treating Type 'A' Behaviour and Your Heart; Meyer Friedman, M.D. and Diana Ulmer, R.N., M.S., Knopf (1984)

Coronary Case; Rex Edwards, Faber paperback (1964)

The Broken Heart, the Medical Consequences of Loneliness; James J. Lynch, Harper & Row (1977)

Coronary Heart Disease and Patterns of Living; Angela Finlayson & James McEwen, Croom Helm (1977)

Heart Attacks Understood; Dr Alan Anderson, Pan (1981)

Your Body doesn't lie; John Diamond, M.D., Warner Books

The Healing Heart; Norman Cousins, International Journal of Cardiology (1983)

STRESS

Social Causes of Illness; Richard Totman, Souvenir Press (1979)

Real Health, the ill effects of stress & their prevention; Alex Poteliakhoff & Malcolm Carruthers, David Poynter Ltd.

Stress without Distress; Hans Selye, Teach Yourself Books, Hodder & Stoughton (1974)

Stress – How to stop your mind killing your body; Walter McQuade & Ann Aikman, Arrow Books (1978)

Stress and the Art of Biofeedback; Barbara B. Brown, Bantam Books (1978)

How to cope with stress; Dr Peter Tyrer, Sheldon Press (1980)

The Stress of Life; Hans Selye, M.D., McGraw Hill (1956)

When I Say No, I Feel Guilty; Manuel J. Smith, Bantam (1975)

Don't say 'yes' when you want to say 'no'; Herbert Fensterheim, Ph.D. and Jean Baer, Futura (1976)

DIET

Jane Brody's Nutrition Book; Bantam Books (1982)
Good Hearted Cookery – Champney's/Slimmer Magazine Guide to Low Cholesterol Cookery; Diane Earnshaw
Eat Your Way to Health; Vicki Peterson, Penguin
The F-Plan Diet; Audrey Eyton

SEX

For women:
The Hite Report; Shere Hite
My Secret Garden; Nancy Friday
For men:
Men & Sex: A Guide to Sexual Fulfilment; Souvenir
How to Make Love to a Woman; Michael Morgenshaw, Pan
For both:
The Pleasure Bond; Masters & Johnson
Treat Yourself to Sex; P. Brown & C. Faulder, Penguin (1979)
The New Sex Therapy; Helen Singer-Kaplan
The Joy of Sex; Alex Comfort, Quartet (1975)
The Limits of Sex; Celia Haddon, Michael Joseph (1982)

BODY

Your Body Speaks its Mind; Stanley Keleman
Living Your Dying; Stanley Keleman
On Death & Dying; Elizabeth Kubler Ross
Depression and The Body; Alexander Lowen
Getting Well Again; Carl & Stephanie Simonton
The Relaxation Response; H. Benson, Morrow, N. York (1975)

CREATIVITY & MEANING

On Not Being Able to Paint; Joanna Field
Man's Search for Meaning; Victor Frankl, Hodder & Stoughton

GENERAL PSYCHOLOGY

On Aggression; Konrad Lorenz
The Undiscovered Self; C. G. Jung
Synchronicity, The Way of Individuation; Jolande Jacobi

BOOKS TO READ

Toward a Psychology of Being; Abraham Maslow
The Inner World of Choice; Frances Wickes, Coventure
The Meaning of Anxiety; Rollo May
To Have or To Be; Erich Fromm
The I and the Not-I; M. Esther Harding, Coventure
The Will to Live; Arnold A. Hutschnacker, M.D., Cornerstone
    Library
Man and His Symbols; C. G. Jung

GENERAL

The Courage to Be; Paul Tillich, Fontana
The Male Menopause; Derek Bowshill & Anthea Linacre, Pan
The Middle Age Crisis; Barbara Fried, Harper & Row (1976)
Powers of Mind; Adam Smith
The Seasons of a Man's Life; Daniel S. Levinson
Passages; Gail Sheehy
Loneliness; Irma Kurtz
Dreams: God's Forgotten Language; John A. Sanford
Dreams and Healing; John A. Sanford
The Diseases of Civilisation; Brian Inglis, Hodder & Stoughton
Gift From The Sea; Anne Morrow Lindbergh, Vintage Books
An Experiment with Time; J. M. Dunne, Papermac
If You Meet the Buddha on the Road, Kill Him; Sheldon Kopp
Mirror, Mask & Shadow; Sheldon Kopp
Journeys of Nothing in the Land of Everything; Eduard Matchett

YOGA & MEDITATION

Mind as Healer, Mind as Slayer; K. R. Pelletier, Delta
Conversations with a Siddha; Swami Muhtananda, SYDA Foundation
Stalking the Wild Pendulum: on the Mechanics of Consciousness; Itzhak
    Benton, Fontana
The Probability of the Impossible; Melina Mons
—HOW TO MEDITATE
Yoga; Ernest Wood, Pelican (1962)

EXERCISE

Jogging; William Bowerman & W. E. Harris MD, Corgi (1968)

HOLISTIC HEALTH

Acupuncture, its place in western medicine; George T. Lewith, Thorsons
Homeopathy & natural medicine; Dr. C. H. Sharma, Turnstone Press (1975)
The Science of Homeopathy; George Vithoulkas, Grove Press, Inc. (1980)
Imagery in Healing; Jeanne Achterberg, New Science Library (1985)
Holistic Health; Lawrence le Shan, Trunstone Press (1985)
Love Your Disease – It's keeping you healthy; John Harrison, Angus & Robertson (1984)

Useful Addresses

The British Holistic Medical Association
179 Gloucester Place
London
NW1 6DX

Write for information about doctors practising holistic medicine.

International Society for Humanism in Cardiology
43 Weymouth Street,
London W1
Tel: 01-486 4191

Write for information and literature.

British Heart Foundation
102 Gloucester Place,
London W1H 4DH

Involved in research into heart disease. Write for pamphlets, medical
and research reports and information about emergency pacemaker
centres and heart attack resuscitation card.

Chest, Heart & Stroke Association
Tavistock House North,
Tavistock Square,
London WC1

Similar to the above. Write for details of their organisation and
literature.

COUNSELLING

British Association for Counselling
1a Little Church Street,
Rugby,
Warwickshire

Write for information about counsellors in your area who are also members. Also booklets on useful topics.

National Marriage Guidance
(Local offices)

See your local telephone directory.

Centre for Transpersonal Psychology
7 Pembridge Place
London W2

Write for information about workshops and counsellors.

Westminster Pastoral Foundation
23 Kensington Square,
London W8
Tel: 01-937 6956

Family counselling service. Write or telephone for information.

GENERAL

Citizens' Advice Bureaux
Head Office: 11 Drury Lane, London WC2
            Tel: 01-836 9231

See local telephone directory.

Health Services Ombudsman
Church House,
Great Smith Street,
London SW1 3BW
Tel: 01-212 7676

USEFUL ADDRESSES

Patients' Association
11 Dartmouth Street,
London SW1
Tel: 01-222 4992

British Red Cross Society
Head Office: 9 Grosvenor Crescent, London SW1
            Tel: 01-235 5454

See local telephone directory. Courses, medical work, first aid
courses.

St. John Ambulance
1 Grosvenor Crescent,
London SW1X 7EF
Tel: 01-235 5231

First aid training and courses.

RELAXATION & MEDITATION

Relaxation for Living
29 Burwood Park Road,
Walton-on-Thames,
Surrey

Transcendental Meditation
Roydon Hall,
Seven Mile Lane,
East Peckham,
Near Tonbridge,
Kent

Write for information about your local T.M. centre where you can
learn meditation techniques.

Centre for Autogenic Training
14a Milford House,
7 Queen Anne Street,
London W1M 9FD
Tel: 01-637 1586

Write for information about courses (usually one a week for eight weeks) to learn their relaxation technique.

Siddha Meditation Centre West One
14a Milford House,
7 Queen Anne Street,
London W1

The Wrekin Trust
Dove House,
Little Birch,
Hereford HR2 8BB
Tel: 0981 540224

Write for list of courses, lectures, literature, taped talks on personal development subjects.

Index

INDEX